I0090807

BEYOND BEAUTY

Proven Secrets to Age Well,
Look 10 Years Younger &
Live a Truly Happy, Healthy, Long Life

Dr. Debbie M. Palmer
with Valerie A. Latona

ISBN 13: **9780692140338**

To my husband and soul mate, Sergio; my children, Matthew and Michael; and my mother with boundless gratitude.

In loving memory of my father and grandparents.

Contents

Introduction

Do you want to look years younger—and have plenty of energy and enthusiasm to keep up with your busy life?

Then you've come to the right place. You've already taken the first step toward change just by picking up this book. Now, stick with me as I guide you through the very doable steps toward radiant, beautiful skin—and a healthy body, spirit, and mind—all of which I detail throughout each chapter of this book.

But first, I'd like you to step back and look in the mirror. Write down the things you'd like to tweak, be it dark under-eye circles; fine lines and wrinkles; dark spots; dull, lackluster skin; dry, rough skin; acne; skin rashes; or whatever it is that you want to improve.

Even better, if you can, take a selfie to record your current look, as a reminder of what you want to change. (This picture will also become your "before" picture in your very own beauty and life makeover.)

What about your weight and your overall health? Is your body performing at its best, or are you often fatigued and frequently getting sick? Take note of how your body feels today—and where you want to be.

Also, be sure to include how you feel. Are you experiencing inner turmoil, sadness, or anxiety? Do you wake up every morning with a feeling of happiness or dread when you think about your day? Do you truly love what you do every day? Do you feel fulfilled with your social connections and relationships?

What about your sleep: how much are you getting every night, and do you wake up feeling rested and recharged? How about your energy levels: do you feel lively or sluggish?

And how's your outlook on life? What are your recurrent thoughts? Are they positive? Are you satisfied with your spiritual connection? Do you take time to slow down and connect with your inner or higher self?

Write everything down—and write down your reason, too, for wanting to change it; these words will be important motivation to keep you on track through this process of inner growth and outer transformation and beauty. True beauty is a radiance that comes from a truly healthy inner self.

What I Want to Change about My Body and My Skin

- ____
- ____
- ____
- ____
- ____

Now, take a habit inventory and see if those things that you're frequently doing are benefitting you. When you're under stress, do you overeat or binge eat, eat unhealthy junk food, smoke, have repetitive negative thoughts, show anger toward others, or fight with loved ones?

Write down the healthy habits you've been meaning to incorporate into your life—but haven't had a chance to do so. Be sure to write the reason you want to incorporate these healthy habits.

Healthy Habits I Want to Incorporate into My Life

- ____
- ____
- ____
- ____
- ____

The reason I have you write down both healthy habits and the things you want to change about your body and skin is that the two are connected. A healthy body equals radiant, glowing skin. I'm sure you've heard it before, but this book will take you through exactly why the two are linked and the specific steps you can take to make all the things you listed above a reality.

Throughout the course of this book, I'll work with you at replacing unhealthy habits with healthy ones. For example, when under stress, instead of turning to your usual ways, maybe you'll take a short walk to blow off steam or sit quietly in a chair for ten minutes and close your eyes and meditate. Or maybe just turning your mind to positive thoughts and giving thanks for the positive things in your life will help. It isn't easy to stop bad habits, but it's easier to replace them with healthy ones. By the end of this book, the healthy choices will become habit!

A good mantra to write down and repeat, as you move through your journey to a healthier, happier, and younger-looking you: "I know that old, negative patterns—of eating, living, working—no longer limit me."

➔Exactly How This Book Will Help You

Everyone these days, it seems, is searching for a quick-fix fountain of youth. I know this because, as a practicing dermatologist in New York for over sixteen years, I get every request imaginable when people walk through the doors of my practice. Patients want to erase years from their skin in minutes so they can walk out looking younger—and be more confident. And while this *is* possible with all the office procedures available in a dermatologist's arsenal today, there's a key component of the aging process that many people are missing out on. And that's a healthy lifestyle.

What you're putting *into* your body—and doing *to* your body on a daily basis—is as critical to the skin-aging process as what you're slathering on or injecting from the outside.

In fact, I would argue that it's even more important.

As one of just several hundred dermatologists in the country trained in osteopathic medicine—a holistic philosophy and approach that relates each part of the body to the entire system—I know that what we do to our bodies on a daily basis affects how much energy we have, our outlook on life, how confident we are—and, yes, how we look on the outside.

I'm confident about what truly works to help people bring change into their lives and look and feel better, because I've seen the results in so many people—of different ages, lifestyles, and cultures—whom I've treated. In my private practice, I've helped thousands of clients learn how to live a healthier, more peaceful and spiritually aware, more productive, more beautiful life.

The skin is a living, functioning organ. In fact, it's the largest organ in the body. Whatever you do to your body, you do to your skin. What I find fascinating is that researchers from the University of Southern Denmark found that the skin actually communicates with the liver,[1] which is the organ in the body that filters out toxins. This explains why if something's going on inside our body, it's often reflected on the skin (rashes, eczema, wrinkles, sallow skin, etc.). I believe this is proof why taking a holistic approach to health and our body, like the one I'm recommending in this book, is so important.

There's a quote I love about the earth by the Indian Chief Seattle that holds true for our body and our skin:

> *"Humankind has not woven the web of life. We are but one thread within it. Whatever we do to the web, we do to ourselves. All things are bound together. All things connect."*

Borrowing from Chief Seattle, I'm going to apply this quote to the body—and skin—and say:

> *"Our skin is but one thread in the aging process. Whatever we do to our bodies, we do to our skin. All things in the body are bound together. All things connect."*

Kate's Story

Take Kate*, for example. Kate is a patient of mine who was beyond stressed in her high-pressure Wall Street finance job. She had put on about ten pounds over the last couple of years, due to on-the-go eating, plenty of travel, not so much sleep, and no time for regular exercise—not to mention practically nonexistent "me" time. She came to me to help her look younger and was requesting several procedures. Not only did Kate look tired and worn out, she also looked ten years older than she actually was. She had dark circles under her eyes, her skin looked dull, and her wrinkles were pronounced.

I discussed in-office procedures with her, but we also talked about the other important elements of beauty that she wasn't paying attention to in her daily life—diet, sleep, stress reduction, a home-maintenance skin-care routine, spirituality, and healthy relationships. All are important elements of beauty—both inside out and outside in.

Kate is not unique. So many of us live lifestyles dictated by stressful, high-powered jobs that leave little time for the key components of healthy living, such as:

- ✓ Eating a diet rich in whole, unprocessed foods (including colorful fruits and vegetables)
- ✓ Drinking plenty of water
- ✓ Taking time out to relax mentally *and* physically
- ✓ Exercising every day
- ✓ Getting enough restful sleep
- ✓ Learning to develop a passion for life again
- ✓ Nurturing healthy relationships
- ✓ Spiritual enrichment

In this book, I'm going to talk about ways to slowly and gradually balance out your life so you're healthier—and your skin looks years younger. You'll have a more positive outlook on life, too, because there's a genuine happiness that comes when all parts of your body are working together in harmony.

Want proof? Next time you go to the grocery store, take a look at what's in people's shopping carts. What you'll find: those with the carts filled with plenty of fruits and vegetables, whole grains like oatmeal, lean (unprocessed) meats, fish, and beans—*not* processed foods, soda, sugar-laden sweets, and unhealthy snack foods—are the ones who have more youthful, radiant skin. They also look and act younger. You might argue that these foods cost more money—and that these people are probably also getting pricey facials and treatments at the dermatologist's office. But healthy eating and healthy living do *not* have to cost a lot of money, as I'll show you in this book. Not eating healthy costs a lot, too. In fact, I'd say that eating an unhealthy diet costs even more: an unhealthy body, a lack of energy (and enthusiasm, as food affects mood), and skin that's not looking its best.

I know the link between nutrition and beauty firsthand. My mother was a dietician when I was growing up and stressed the importance of vitamins and minerals in food choices. This influenced me to take a nutrition course in graduate school—and I was hooked from that point on. I realized that the food we eat every day is such an important part of overall well-being.

I also realized how vitamins, minerals, and particularly antioxidants (key substances—often nutrients—that fight disease-causing and aging molecules in the body called free radicals) fit into our lives and keep us healthy. I continued to study nutrition, and particularly antioxidants, through medical school and have incorporated the healthy habits detailed in this book into my own life. I also recommend these healthy Beyond Beauty strategies to each of my patients.

In fact, osteopathy—one type of medicine practiced commonly by primary-care doctors throughout America and some dermatologists like myself—is a holistic, preventive approach to medicine that believes each part of the body, including the skin, is connected to the entire system.

Something that's important to know about me: I'm not against aging but *for* aging well. I had my children later in life (in my forties), so I'm motivated to take care of myself and stay healthy, energetic, and youthful so I can enjoy my family for years to come. And having enough energy and vitality to enjoy every day of our lives is something we all can accomplish—by putting into practice the essential tools and information in this book.

The Difference Between a DO and an MD

When you think of a doctor, you most likely assume that they have an MD (which stands for Medical Doctor) after their name—but not all doctors do. Some, like me, have a DO (which stands for Doctor of Osteopathy) after their name. Here's a breakdown of the similarities and differences between an MD and a DO:

Education: Both a DO and an MD have 4-year medical degrees and complete a residency of 3 to 7 years.

Treatment: Both a DO and an MD utilize scientifically accepted methods of diagnosis and treatment, including the use of prescription drugs and surgery.

Philosophy of care: This is where a DO and an MD may differ. The osteopathic philosophy focuses on a holistic approach to practicing medicine—meaning DOs treat the patient as a whole, not just their symptoms or injuries. (Keep in mind that some MDs do this as well, but they're not *trained* to do so.) Osteopathic medicine also places emphasis on prevention of disease, though some MDs are starting to adopt this philosophy as well. Traditionally, Medical Doctors practice the classical form of medicine focused on the diagnosis and treatment of disease.

It's not easy, though. Having radiant, youthful skin and a healthy body takes hard work and commitment, but if you follow these secrets of aging well—eating healthy food; managing stress, thinking positive, and connecting to your inner spiritual self; exercising regularly; getting enough sleep; and using proven strategies to rejuvenate the skin—you'll be able to age gracefully, feel and look years younger, and live longer.

All I ask is that you don't give up; stick with me through this entire process—and throughout each chapter of this book—and you will see change, guaranteed. One of my favorite motivational thoughts is:

"Each day is a new opportunity. Yesterday is done. Today is the first day of my future."

Make this saying your motivational motto as you journey on this path toward inner and outer beauty.

How to Age Well in the Modern World

To get started, I want to ask: How old would you be if you didn't know how old you were?

If we all were to sit down and think about this, we would realize that our age is so much more than the number of wrinkles we have on our skin or the number of candles on a birthday cake. It's the state of our health, how we feel, how much energy we have, and how happy and confident we are each and every day now—and throughout every moment of our journey. In the wise words of Betty Friedan:

> *"Aging is not lost youth, but a new stage of opportunity and strength."*

In a nutshell, how old we are is a result of how we treat our bodies every day: how much we sleep, what we eat, how we cope with stress, whether we exercise or not, how positive we are—about ourselves, our relationships, and our life—and, of course, how we care for our skin. Our skin and the fine lines, wrinkles, and other signs of aging that we see when we look in the mirror are just the icing on the proverbial age cake. But it's the entire holistic picture of our body—and our health, both physical and emotional—that contributes to how old we truly are and how long and well we'll live.

I know this firsthand. As a busy mom of two, I know that eating healthy foods, exercising regularly, getting enough sleep, and spending time meditating (even if it's just five or ten minutes a day) helps me stay balanced and get everything I need to get done, done. It also helps me avoid getting sick with every cold and illness that my kids bring home from school. This healthy lifestyle keeps me sane, too, particularly when work and my personal life get crazy busy at the same time (which happens a lot!).

Let me share a personal story: Just recently, I accompanied my older son to a Boy Scout camp for the weekend. We spent the weekend tubing, hiking, climbing ropes and rock walls, and generally staying active the entire time. I was able to keep up, I know, because I try to follow a healthy lifestyle most days. When I don't, I can feel it: I'm sluggish and have low energy. Sure, there are times when I have pizza or indulge in some chocolate or potato chips, but moderation is key to everything. I use the 80/20 rule: 80 percent of the time, I make sure to really try to do everything right for my body, and 20 percent of the time, I let myself indulge or skip a workout if I'm really busy. No one can be perfect!

In fact, this book isn't about being perfect. It's about making small tweaks in your daily routine that equal big changes in your life, your health, your skin, and your longevity.

In each of the sections that follow, I'll be giving you practical tips and advice for your daily life, based on the very latest scientific evidence and research, on how to be well...so you can age well, ward off debilitating illness and disease, be happy, have a healthy mental outlook, and have enough energy to do all the things you want to do—and look gorgeous every step of the way.

CHAPTER 1

Give Your Diet a Mediterranean Makeover

"Tell me what you eat, and I will tell you what you are."

~ *Jean Anthelme Brillat-Savarin*

One of my patients, Samantha*, has been troubled by adult acne for over twenty years. She came to see me because she had tried other treatments that just weren't bringing her long-term relief. We talked about the treatments that were right for her, such as topical acne medications, but we also addressed some critical aspects to healthy skin, including her diet and her lifestyle (including stress reduction).

It turned out that Samantha drank a lot of diet soda every day and regularly ate fast food and drank alcohol. She tweaked her diet, cutting down on soda and alcohol and opting for fresh, nutrient-rich whole foods instead of takeout.

Samantha also started taking Vinyasa yoga to reduce her stress, and she swapped out her makeup and moisturizer for noncomedogenic (non-pore-clogging) options.

The result: Samantha's skin cleared up—and stayed acne free. She developed a healthy glow, and she began to look years younger. She recently told me that she feels like a new person and gets compliments all the time on how great she looks. "At my age," she told me, "my skin has never looked better!"

Like Samantha, patient after patient in my practice tells me that when they follow my advice about eating a healthy diet, their skin is transformed. No, it doesn't happen overnight, but it does happen. Acne is cleared up. Rashes and eczema disappear. Dry skin becomes more hydrated. Skin becomes more radiant and youthful looking.

I remind patients to treat their skin as one very important part of their whole being. Every aspect of our body (including the skin) works together; when one part of the body is out of balance, it shows up on the skin. And then, when the body is out of balance for long periods of time, whole-body illness and disease sets in—and eventually, our longevity is affected.

Consider it this way: the skin—one of the largest organs in the body—is a very important part of our whole body. In fact, problems on the skin can be the very first sign that something's out of balance with the rest of our body.

So what diet do I recommend to all my patients (and follow myself)? No, not juice fasts, raw-vegetable-only diets, or restrictive calorie diets. What I recommend: a Mediterranean style of eating, which is healthy and delicious, and the benefits of which have been proven over hundreds of years. The benefits of this style of eating and living go way beyond the skin—feeding what I like to say is truly beauty, and health, from the inside out.

What Is the Mediterranean Diet?

Did you know that the Japanese people—particularly those from the southern Japanese Okinawa islands—have the highest proportion of centenarians (a person who lives to or beyond one hundred years of age) in the world?[2] And within these islands, Ogimi—a tiny village—has more than a dozen centenarians! These people have been studied, and experts have determined that it's not just their leisurely way of life that contributes to their longevity. It's what—and how—they eat, namely a garden-to-table diet that is so similar to the Mediterranean style of eating, with their fruits and vegetables coming straight from their own backyards and their fresh fish coming out of the ocean that morning, bypassing the middleman and the fish farms that are so common today.

We've heard the term "Mediterranean diet" talked about, but it's not a specific diet plan or miracle cleanse that will help you magically drop pounds. It's more of a collection of eating habits—or a style of eating—that's followed by the sixteen countries bordering the Mediterranean Sea, including Greece, Southern Italy, and Spain.[3] (It's also very similar to our modern-day DASH diet, which stands for Dietary Approaches to Stop Hypertension.)

The Mediterranean diet is high in olive oil, fish, legumes, fresh fruit (typically as a daily dessert), nuts, unrefined cereals (like bran cereal), and fresh vegetables, along with moderate consumption of dairy (mostly as cheese and yogurt), poultry, and wine—and low in red meat. Because of its composition, it's also a diet low in saturated fat and high in mono- and polyunsaturated fat and dietary fiber.

For these reasons, it has numerous health benefits, ranging from cardiovascular-disease prevention to a lower risk of cancer. In fact, people who eat this type of diet high in polyunsaturated fats—which come from fish and plants—are less likely to die from heart disease or *any* cause.[4]

One study in particular found that people—in this case Midwestern firefighters—who followed this Mediterranean style of eating (like those on the Greek island of Ikaria) had lower risk factors for cardiovascular disease.[5] This research found specifically that the firefighters with the greatest adherence to a Mediterranean-style diet showed a 35 percent decreased risk in something called the metabolic syndrome—a condition with risk factors that include a large waistline, high triglyceride level, low HDL ("good") cholesterol level, high blood pressure, and high blood sugar. They also had a 43 percent lower risk of weight gain.

This diet also seems to lower cardiovascular risk by lowering levels of unhealthy blood triglycerides[6]—associated with an increased risk of hardening of the arteries. Another study found that this style of eating is associated with a lower prevalence of obesity (a risk factor for heart disease and even breast cancer).[7]

Take a look at this Mediterranean food pyramid for more specifics:

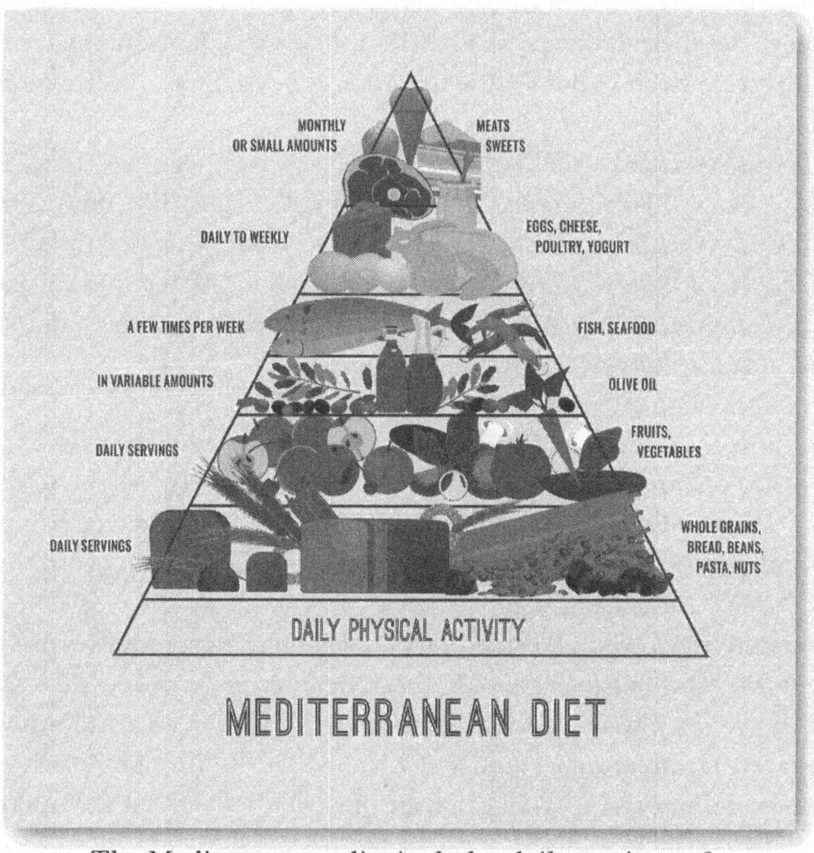

The Mediterranean diet includes daily servings of whole grains, beans, nuts/seeds, and fruits and vegetables. Healthy fats like olive oil are also important.

Their diet is super fresh and chock-full of what I like to call longevity food and nutrients—key nutrients that keep your body humming along at its healthiest and your skin at its radiant best. They also consume three servings of fresh fish a week (including squid and octopus—both rich in protein, nutrients, and stay-healthy antioxidants like taurine), plenty of whole grains (like barley, bulgur wheat, and steel-cut oats), and indigenous vegetables like seaweed. These color-dense vegetables (like purple and orange sweet potatoes) are grown without the use of pesticides and are rich in a variety of nutrients including antioxidants such as flavonoids, carotenoids, vitamin E, and lycopene. The Okinawans also eat plenty of legumes: lentils, chickpeas, pinto beans, and white and black beans—as well as drinking plenty of antioxidant-rich green tea.

On Okinawa, people also practice something called "hara hachi bu," which means eating moderately and only to 80 percent fullness. They believe the other 20 percent will only go to enrich doctors.[8] This is something I put into practice in my own life: I try not to eat to extreme fullness, because it's uncomfortable and because I know it's just not healthy for you. In fact, eating small, frequent meals—and not large meals that can trigger this uncomfortable fullness—is best. Small, frequent meals (eaten slowly and mindfully) don't tax the digestive system and create fewer free radicals in the body (more on free radicals later on in this chapter).

And then there's the Greek island of Ikaria, called "The Island Where People Forget to Die."[9] Ikarian men are nearly four times as likely as their American counterparts to reach the age of ninety. They also live about eight to ten years longer before succumbing to cancers and cardiovascular disease—and they suffer less depression and about a quarter the rate of dementia.

The Ikarians' diet plays a big part in this, say experts like Christina Chrysohoou, MD, a cardiologist at the University of Athens School of

Medicine, who conducted a study of almost seven hundred Ikarians.[10] She found that these Ikarians eat a Mediterranean diet—consuming about six times as many beans a day as Americans, eating fish twice a week and meat five times a month (typically from their own livestock), drinking about two to three cups of coffee a day, and eating much less refined sugar.

This cardiologist also discovered that these island peoples consumed high levels of olive oil, along with two to four glasses of red wine a day. They also regularly ate wild greens (from their own pesticide-free gardens), which have ten times as many antioxidants as red wine. The Ikarians are also known to drink a daily local mountain tea made from antioxidant-rich dried herbs like marjoram, sage, and rosemary.

This type of vegetable-based diet—along with moderate amounts of antioxidant-rich red wine—contributes not just to how long you live, but to the vitality in those years. It helps keep you happy, radiant, energetic, and mobile, without aches and pains, and it helps prevent your mind from deteriorating as it does with dementia and Alzheimer's.

One study in particular found that a diet rich in dark, leafy green vegetables, beans, berries, whole grains, and red wine—the very diet of the Ikarians and Okinawans—can actually slow normal brain aging and cognitive decline.[11] The study, conducted by the Rush University Medical Center in Chicago, was based on something called the MIND diet (which stands for Mediterranean-DASH Diet Intervention for Neurodegenerative Delay). Followers of this diet limited the kinds of foods common in an American diet but not eaten in the Ikarian or Okinawan diet: red meat, butter, stick margarine, cheese, pastries and sweets, and fried and fast food.

What's more: the Ikarians—like the Okinawans—take time to relax and enjoy their meals with others, an important health-promoting social aspect. Socializing has been shown in studies to be important for maintaining good mental health[12] and for warding off diseases like dementia, Alzheimer's, and even heart disease.[13] Socializing also promotes happiness—a key factor for inner and outer beauty.

The Many Benefits of a Mediterranean Diet

Like the Ikarians and the Okinawans, if you make at least half your plate fruits and vegetables, you'll get as many good-for-you (and good-for-your-skin) nutrients as possible. You'll also fill up on healthy fiber, which has been shown to help reduce the risk of everything from heart disease and diabetes[14] to kidney stones[15] and constipation. In fact, one study found that people who ate the most fiber were less likely to die of any cause.[16] The average adult only gets about fifteen grams of fiber a day, but women need at least twenty-five grams per day, and men need at least thirty-eight grams daily.

Top sources of fiber include foods found in a Mediterranean diet, such as legumes like peas and beans; whole grains like oatmeal, barley, and brown rice; nuts and seeds; and, of course, fruits and vegetables (if possible, with the peel, as it contains lots of fiber).

There's plenty of research, detailed here, that points to the health benefits of a Mediterranean diet beyond just the nutrients like fiber that it provides. But the main things my patients notice when switching over to this type of diet: more energy; less sickness; weight loss; better sleep; and healthier, more radiant skin.

And when it comes to the research, studies show that this type of Mediterranean diet reduces overall mortality,[17] and reduces your risk of major diseases that can take a toll on your body, your skin, and more.

This is a lot of research, but stick with me on this; this is the core of the science behind the Mediterranean diet—and it proves just how important this way of eating is for health and longevity.

It keeps your heart healthy. Numerous studies have shown the dramatic effects of a Mediterranean diet on heart health. In a landmark Lyon Heart Study, higher ALA (a type of omega-3 healthy fat found in fish, vegetables, and yogurt) consumption—a hallmark of the Mediterranean diet—dramatically reduced total and cardiovascular mortality as well as nonfatal myocardial infarctions by more than 70 percent.[18] Another study, conducted by Greek researchers, showed that adults who closely followed a Mediterranean diet were 47 percent less likely to develop heart disease over a ten-year period than adults who didn't follow this diet closely.[19]

It keeps your brain sharp. Numerous studies have detailed the benefits of a Mediterranean diet for the brain. One study found that people over sixty-five who eat more fish, vegetables, fruit, grains, and olive oil have a larger brain volume than those who don't follow a Mediterranean-style diet.[20] In another study, researchers from Columbia University Medical Center and Washington University reviewed brain MRIs of 712 octogenarians and found that those who followed a diet rich in olive oil, whole grains, fish, vegetables, and fruit were up to 36 percent less likely to show brain damage (associated with cognitive problems) from small strokes.[21] And according to one study in the *Journal of the American Medical Association*, following a Mediterranean diet can reduce the risk of developing Alzheimer's disease by 48 percent, when combined with regular exercise.[22]

It reduces your risk of cancer. Patients who followed a Mediterranean-style diet had reduced mortality from all causes, but also a decreased risk of cancer overall.[23] One study in particular found that eating this Mediterranean-style diet is associated with a significantly lower risk of stomach cancer.[24] Other research, published in the *American Journal of Epidemiology*, found that postmenopausal women who eat a Mediterranean-style diet had a reduced risk of breast cancer.[25] Eating this type of diet also cuts the risk of endometrial cancer in women by 57 percent.[26,27]

This plant-based style of eating may also protect against skin cancer. Mediterranean populations have very low rates of skin cancer—despite living in sunny climates. The incidence of melanomas (the deadliest form of skin cancer) in Mediterranean countries is lower than in Northern Europe and significantly lower in other warm-weather countries like New Zealand and Australia. Some experts theorize that the components of a Mediterranean diet (namely the powerful disease-fighting antioxidants found in it) may provide protection against skin cancer.[28]

It reduces your risk of diabetes. Eating a plant-based diet can help reduce your risk of obesity (which is a top risk factor for type 2 diabetes), but replacing saturated fats (like palm oil, butter, and cheese) with monounsaturated fats—typical of the Mediterranean region, which emphasizes fruits, vegetables, whole grains, legumes, nuts, and olive oil—has been found to improve insulin sensitivity, which may explain, say researchers, "the favorable effect of the Mediterranean diet on glucose and insulin levels."[29] Researchers also found that eating a diet with omega-3 fatty acids (found in the seeds, nuts, and fish prevalent in a Mediterranean diet) also improves insulin sensitivity.[30]

According to researchers,[31] 90 percent of type 2 diabetes (as well as 80 percent of coronary heart disease and 70 percent of strokes) can be avoided by eating a Mediterranean-style diet, getting regular physical activity, and not smoking.[32]

It reduces your risk of developing depression. Research published in the *Archives of General Psychiatry* shows that people who follow a Mediterranean-style of eating are less likely to develop depression.[33] Another study in the *Journal of Public Health Nutrition* found that adequate intake of fruits, nuts, vegetables, unrefined cereals, legumes, and fish (all key components of a Mediterranean diet) provided a variety of nutrients that are important to depression prevention.[34]

It may help protect your kidneys. Adhering to a Mediterranean diet may significantly reduce your risk of developing chronic kidney disease, say researchers.[35] Nine hundred participants were followed for seven years. Those who followed the Mediterranean diet most closely had a 50 percent lower risk of developing chronic kidney disease.

It reduces your risk of Parkinson's disease. Researchers have found that eating plenty of fruit, vegetables, legumes, whole grains, nuts, fish, and poultry, along with a low intake of saturated fat and a moderate intake of alcohol (all of which are characteristics of a Mediterranean diet) may protect against Parkinson's disease[36]—a chronic and progressive movement disorder.

It reduces the symptoms of rheumatoid arthritis. One pilot study of women found that those who followed a Mediterranean diet improved symptoms, disease activity, and cardiovascular risk.[37]

It may help you breathe better. Several studies have found that following a Mediterranean diet helps improve asthmatic symptoms in both children[38] and adults.[39] One study also found that eating a Mediterranean-style diet rich in vegetables, whole grains, polyunsaturated fats like olive oil, and nuts—and low in red and processed meat, refined grains, and sugary drinks—is associated with a lower risk of chronic lung disease.[40]

It reduces your risk of vision problems. A study by the Centre for Eye Research in Australia found that people who consume at least one hundred milliliters (about seven tablespoons) of olive oil a week are almost 50 percent less likely to develop macular degeneration (the most common cause of poor eyesight in older people) than those who eat less than one milliliter (less than one tablespoon) a week.[41]

It keeps your smile healthy. Low doses of omega-3 fatty acids (found in a Mediterranean diet)—namely EPA (eicosapentaenoic acid), DHA (docosahexaenoic acid), and ALA (alpha-linolenic acid) have been found to have strong antibacterial activity in the mouth, inhibiting oral pathogens like *Streptococcus* (strep), *Candida albicans*, and *Porphyromonas ginigivalis*, all of which can trigger gum disease.[42]

~ BEYOND BEAUTY RECIPE ~
Poached Salmon With Lemon Vinaigrette

Salmon is a protein-rich Mediterranean staple, full of omega-3 fatty acids.

Ingredients
For the salmon
1 (4-pound) wild salmon fillet, skin off, cut into 5-ounce portions
2 organic celery stalks, diced
2 organic onions, diced
2 organic carrots, diced
3 bay leaves
2 cups white wine
8 cups water
For the lemon vinaigrette
5 organic garlic cloves, smashed
2 organic shallots, sliced
2 organic lemons, with zest and juice
2 cups white wine
2 tablespoons whole-grain mustard
1 c organic extra virgin olive oil

Pink Himalayan sea salt (rich in vital minerals not found in table salt)
Ground white pepper
2 pounds organic salad greens
1 bunch organic chives, minced

Directions
For salmon Place ingredients in stockpot, and simmer 15 to 20 minutes. Strain stock; season with salt, pepper. In roasting pan, bring stock to simmer. Submerge salmon in stock; cook to desired doneness (about 20 minutes). Remove salmon with spatula. Chill until ready to eat. *For lemon vinaigrette* Place garlic, shallots, lemon zest, and white wine in pot over medium heat. Allow wine to reduce to half. Add salt, pepper, and juice of lemon. Chill. Add mixture into blender, add mustard; blend until smooth. Drizzle in olive oil. *For assembly* Toss greens with vinaigrette. Place salmon on salad, drizzle with vinaigrette; garnish with minced chives.

How an Island Diet Translates to Modern Life

If you look at the diet of these island populations, it's easy to see that food is where everything begins: it nourishes us, provides us energy, makes us healthy (or establishes the groundwork for illness and disease), gives a glow (or dull cast) to our skin, and can prolong our lives (or shorten them).

We know inherently what's good for us—what we *should* be eating: more fruits and vegetables, healthy whole grains, protein, healthy fats (as compared with the unhealthy fried ones), low sugar and sodium, fewer unhealthy carbohydrates, plenty of water (not soda), and no junk.

But as much as we *know* about good nutrition, it's so very complicated (and hard, I know) to put this healthy way of eating into practice in our modern society. Long work days, after-school and weekend children's activities, lack of time to prepare healthy foods, the 24/7 availability of unhealthy convenience foods, sugar cravings (mindless munching), fatigue, and few to no backyard gardens to supply all our produce needs—all factor into why eating a healthy diet isn't so easy in our daily lives. But food is the foundation for health and beauty; that is why I start this book here.

I want to share the story of my grandmother. When I was young, she was overweight and had high blood pressure and cholesterol. She never had a lot of energy to really do much (this I remember so well). She was sedentary and tired most of the time and would quickly lose her breath with exertion.

But then something changed. I remember her telling me that her doctor spoke to her about the benefits of eating healthy—with more fruits and vegetables—and exercising. She spent time reading about these topics and would tell me about the things she learned. I would visit her on weekends, and we would prepare the family meals together. While we were cooking together, she would tell me about the benefits of various ingredients we were using—and why they were healthy for me.

This was where I first heard about the benefits of avocados, tomatoes, and bananas. Along with eating healthy, my grandparents turned their den into an exercise room with a stationary bike, rowing machine, and treadmill. Then her body transformed: she lost a lot of weight, and I know, from talking to her as I got older, that she decreased her blood pressure and cholesterol medications. She felt better, had more energy, and was more mobile. She wanted to do things. She was happy. She also exuded radiance and beauty as she began to enjoy life again. This made a huge impression on me—and is something that I think about with my own children.

Bottom line: healthy eating and exercise and treating our bodies right make such a huge difference—and for some people, may even allow them to decrease or go off medications, like my grandmother did.

The wrong foods trigger inflammation throughout the body, and the right foods nourish us, quelling this inflammation.

Numerous studies have pointed to this systemic—or body-wide—inflammation as one of the leading triggers for premature aging (in the body and on the skin) and a leading cause of chronic diseases: cardiovascular disease, type 2 diabetes, Alzheimer's disease, and many types of cancer.[43] And numerous studies, including one published in the *Journal of the American College of Cardiology*,[44] have found that a healthy, whole-foods diet—often referred to as a Mediterranean diet—reduces inflammation. Another study backed this up, saying that specifically the Mediterranean and Okinawan diets help reduce inflammation and cardiovascular risk.[45] I cite these studies here, and throughout the book, so you can see firsthand the research that's been done to back up the importance of this type of diet for your health.

Combine These Foods for Better Health

There's increasing proof that what you eat is as important as what you combine it with. In fact, one study, published in the *American Journal of Clinical Nutrition*, found that eating the right combination of foods (e.g., fish and vegetables) can help you lose weight, while the wrong combination (e.g., red meat and white bread) can contribute to weight gain.[46]

Some healthy food combinations include:

Tomatoes and broccoli. In one University of Illinois study, eating tomatoes and broccoli together was shown to be better at fighting cancer than each individual food was alone.[47]

Tomatoes and avocados. Fats make carotenoids more bioavailable (which means that the body is better able to use them). And as I mentioned earlier, adding olive oil (another healthy fat) to pasta sauce—a Mediterranean staple—makes the antioxidants in the pasta sauce more available to the body.

Strawberries and grapes. Well, actually, eating a variety of antioxidant-rich fruits (they don't have to be these two) gives you a more powerful antioxidant punch.[48] The idea is that you don't have to limit yourself to one or two: make a fruit salad, and you'll get even more health-protective benefits.

Green tea, dark chocolate, and apples. This makes a healthy afternoon snack, because research shows that the catechins (powerful polyphenols, or antioxidants) in green tea and chocolate work synergistically with quercetin (a flavonoid or another powerful antioxidant) found in apples and onions. Together, they work to loosen clumpy blood platelets, improving cardiovascular health.[49]

Curry and black pepper. Research shows that turmeric (a key component of curry)—which has powerful anti-inflammatory benefits—is better absorbed when combined with black pepper.[50]

I'm also a big believer in combining healthy vegetables, grains, and a plant-based protein—something that's put into practice every day in the Mediterranean cultures. It's simply easier to digest—and healthier too!

Chronic Inflammation and Your Health

Inflammation is actually the core of our body's healing and immune response. When something harmful or irritating affects a part of our body, an inflammatory cascade of events is set in motion: blood flow increases to that area, and along with it, healing proteins and infection-fighting white blood cells. Without inflammation, wounds and infections would never heal.

As with stress, though, some inflammation is healthy, but chronic inflammation—which some experts describe as an immune-system response that's out of control—is not. An unhealthy diet is one of the key triggers of inflammation. A Mediterranean diet, however, can nourish your body and skin with the right nutrients and prevent (or even quell) chronic inflammation, contributing to a more youthful body and more radiant, glowing, and healthy (aka more youthful-looking) skin.

➔How Inflammation Wreaks Havoc on Your Skin

Our skin is a reflection of our total body health. This is something that I talk about with my patients when they come into see me. A nutritious diet that keeps our inside healthy will help keep our outward appearance looking healthy, and the opposite is true in that a poor diet will also show up on our skin.

Inflammation has been called "Skin Enemy Number One"[51] for good reason. It's been linked to skin problems like rosacea, eczema, and psoriasis. In fact, people with inflammatory conditions like eczema have been found to have an increased risk of heart disease and stroke[52]—a possible long-term effect of chronic inflammation within the body.

Inflammation and acne. Inflammation has also been linked to acne. In fact, one study—published in the *Journal of Clinical and Aesthetic Dermatology*[53]—found that systemic inflammation throughout the body can trigger acne breakouts on the skin.[54] Research also shows that people with acne are under increased systemic and skin oxidative stress (defined as a "disturbance" in the balance between the production of harmful free radicals, triggered by stress, and the body's own protective antioxidant defenses)[55]—and appear to consume antioxidants at a faster pace than their acne-free peers.

A good way to improve the health of your skin is to eat foods that regulate your blood-sugar levels. Some foods make your blood sugar rise quickly, triggering your body to make a burst of the hormone insulin to help your cells absorb the sugar. Research suggests that insulin plays a role in acne (causing the growth of pore-clogging cells, an increase in oil production, and inflammatory mediators). I advise patients to keep their blood sugar steady, which fights inflammation and oxidative damage, by following these steps:

(1) Eat foods with a low glycemic index (GI). Glycemic index is a number. It gives you an idea about how fast your body converts the carbohydrates in a food into glucose. The smaller the number, the less impact the food has on your blood sugar:

55 or less = low (good)
56 to 69 = medium
70 or higher = high (bad)

Look for the glycemic index on the labels of packaged foods. You can also find glycemic-index lists for common foods on the Internet.A diet with a lower glycemic load closely follows a Mediterranean diet. This type of diet has:

More	**Fewer**
✓ whole grains	✓ processed foods
✓ nuts	✓ potatoes
✓ legumes	✓ white rice
✓ fruits	✓ pasta
✓ vegetables	✓ white bread
✓ lean protein	✓ sugar

(2) Eat foods close to how they're found in nature. These foods tend to have a lower glycemic index than refined and processed foods.

(3) Eat small meals often. Eating every two to three hours will help keep your blood sugar and insulin levels steadier.

(4) Eat plenty of vegetables, and choose veggies across a range of colors. These will provide a variety of antioxidants that neutralize free-radical damage and inflammation. How you cook your vegetables also makes a difference in which antioxidants you're getting and how much of them you're taking in.

Overcooking vegetables (and fruits) can deplete heat-sensitive nutrients like vitamins C (an antioxidant) and B. If you do have to cook them, one study—published in the *Journal of Agricultural and Food Chemistry*—found that boiling and steaming maintained the antioxidant compounds of vegetables, whereas frying caused a significantly higher loss of antioxidants.[56] Here are some specifics on how to cook certain vegetables to preserve their healthy nutrients:

– **Cooking broccoli.** Researchers found that steaming actually increased broccoli's content of glucosinolates, a group of plant compounds touted for their cancer-fighting abilities. But again, you can't cook broccoli (and other vitamin C–rich foods) for too long; not only will they become wilted, they'll lose important nutrients.

My rule of thumb for cooking is to steam the veggies, and once you can visibly see the steam, turn off the heat and let the steam cook the vegetables. Then check to make sure the vegetables are still bright green (in the case of broccoli) and still slightly crisp. Once they're done, remove the lid and let the steam out.

– **Cooking carrots.** When it comes to carrots, researchers from Newcastle University found that if you cook them whole before cutting them, you can actually boost their nutrient content by 25 percent.[57] The reason: Cut carrots have a higher surface area in contact with the water, say the researchers, resulting in greater loss of nutrients compared with boiling them whole. The heat softens the cell walls in the vegetable, allowing nutrients to leach out.

– **Cooking tomatoes.** Even though you lose vitamin C content through cooking, when cooking tomatoes, you increase the levels of lycopene—a beneficial compound called a phytochemical, a key antioxidant, which makes the tomatoes red. That's according to a team of researchers at Cornell University,[58] who found that cooking tomatoes (as you would with fresh pasta or pizza sauce) enhances their levels of antioxidants. It's also been found that eating olive oil (a key staple of a Mediterranean diet) along with cooked tomatoes helps enhance the absorption of key nutrients.

(5) Drink plenty of water. It's a great way to flush out internal toxins and hydrate your skin from the inside out.

(6) Eat foods high in omega-3s. They've been shown to control the production of leukotriene B_4, a molecule that can increase sebum or oil and cause inflammatory acne. Omega-3s can be found in supplements or in foods like walnuts, avocados, flaxseed oil, and fish like salmon, mackerel, and sardines.

(7) Eat foods high in antioxidants. Antioxidants like vitamins A, C, and E, as well as flavonoids found in red wine, colorful fruits and vegetables, and green tea, all have an anti-inflammatory effect on the skin. Deficiencies in antioxidant minerals such as zinc and selenium have also been linked to acne.

These foods, in particular, are healthy for the skin:

Alfalfa sprouts are packed with anti-inflammatory antioxidants.

Artichokes are a good source of vitamin C, which is found naturally in high amounts in the skin (but which is depleted by things like exposure to the sun's ultraviolet rays).

Avocados are rich in vitamin E and C and can reduce skin inflammation and naturally moisturize the skin.

Broccoli contains vitamins A, B, C, E, and K. These antioxidants fight radical damage and inflammatory skin conditions like acne.

Brown rice is a rich source of vitamin B, protein, magnesium, and several antioxidants. For acne, vitamin B acts as our skin's stress fighter, which helps regulate hormones levels and reduce the likelihood of breakouts.

Garlic is another antioxidant food that helps fight inflammation. It's full of a naturally occurring chemical called allicin, which makes it a potent antibacterial and antiviral.

Nuts contain selenium, vitamin E, copper, magnesium, manganese, potassium, calcium, and iron, which are all important for healthy skin. And while selenium is important for many biological functions like immune response, fertility, and thyroid-hormone production, it's also a powerful antioxidant and natural detoxer—helping get rid of damaging chemicals in the body.[59]

Red grapes contain antioxidants in their fruit and seeds that have been shown to treat inflammatory skin conditions such as psoriasis, eczema, and acne.

And when it comes to antioxidants, I found this tip interesting: adding a hard-boiled egg to your salad (or any raw veggies) will help you absorb more of the critical antioxidants from fresh raw vegetables.[60]

(8) Limit dairy. Studies have found a connection between acne and milk and milk products (e.g., cheese, cream cheese, cottage cheese, ice cream, and even instant breakfast drinks).[61] One reason may be that most of the milk we drink is produced by pregnant cows and contains high levels of hormones that increase oil-gland production. Progesterone, insulin-like growth factor (IGF-1), and compounds that the human body turns into dehydrotestosterone (DHT) are in the milk, which can aggravate acne.

(9) Limit soy consumption. It's been linked to acne. There are natural plant estrogens found in soybeans. Phytoestrogens mimic human estrogen, and that can throw off our hormones.

(10) Get enough probiotics. These healthy bacteria—found in everything from yogurt and kefir to fermented foods—have been found to help acne. One study found that stress, anxiety, and depression can trigger altered gut flora, essentially an overgrowth of unhealthy bacteria in the gut.[62] This overgrowth then leads to inflammation in the body and triggers manifestations in the skin like acne.

But getting enough probiotics (which helps balance the gut) seems to improve acne, as well as increasing production of ceramides in the skin (these are lipid molecules found on the surface layer of the skin) and restoring skin's barrier function, which is essentially the body's ability to keep out the bad stuff (like chemicals, bacteria, and sunlight) and keep in the good stuff (like moisture).

Why Bacteria Keep You Healthy

Our bodies are pretty active petri dishes. There's a mix of good and bad bacteria living inside each of us from our skin (a few hundred species have been identified on the skin[63]) to our intestines.

In fact, it's been estimated that the human body is composed 10 percent of human cells and 90 percent of bacteria.[64] Human cells are outnumbered thirty-three to one! That means there could be trillions of bacteria inside our bodies. It's no wonder the body with all these microorganisms is often referred to as "the human microbiome."

Nowhere is this more evident than in the gut. Bacteria line the intestines and help you digest food. During this process of digestion, they make essential vitamins, send signals to the immune system, and create small molecules that can help your brain function properly. Some studies also indicate that these gut microbes may even affect our circadian rhythm—the internal body clock that regulates almost every part of the body, including sleep—and metabolism.[65]

The research: Researchers have determined that adding healthy bacteria to our bodies—through diet or supplements—can help reduce gas and bloating and increase regularity.

– **Probiotics and metabolic syndrome:** Healthy gut bacteria can also help treat or prevent something called metabolic syndrome—a combination of risk factors that increase a person's chances of getting cardiovascular disease, diabetes, and stroke.[66] People with metabolic syndrome are twice as likely to develop heart disease and five times as likely to develop diabetes as the general population, according to the National Institutes of Health.

– Probiotics and mood: Recent research has found that healthy bacteria in the gut are also responsible for the production of the feel-good chemical serotonin.[67] Since serotonin is a critical neurotransmitter in the body (meaning it helps send nerve messages back and forth along the nerve pathways of the body), it's always been associated with the nervous system. What's fascinating is that now, it's estimated that 90 percent of the body's serotonin is made in the digestive tract. What that means: a healthy digestive system, with the right balance of bacteria, can make a huge difference in relaxation levels and mood, as well as the overall regeneration of cells—another key role of serotonin in the body.

– BEYOND BEAUTY RECIPE –
Kimchi

This popular Korean pickled dish is made by mixing cabbage with seasonings and then allowing it to ferment—a process that gives it its powerful probiotic benefits.

Ingredients
1 organic Napa cabbage head
3 Tbsp pink Himalayan sea salt
1 medium daikon (organic, if possible)
1 organic carrot, shredded
½ cup organic scallions
½ organic apple
1 Tbsp organic ginger, peeled
½ organic red bell pepper, diced
6 organic garlic cloves
3 Tbsp Asian fish sauce
3 Tbsp organic brown rice flour
1 c Korean kimchi pepper flakes

Directions
Chop the head of cabbage into 1-inch by 2-inch strips (the length of the whole cabbage head). Place into a large bowl and mix in salt; set aside. Combine the kimchi mix: julienne the daikon, carrots, and scallions, and place into a large mixing bowl. In a blender, place the sliced apple (cored and peeled) and add the rice flour, peeled ginger, garlic, diced bell pepper, and fish sauce.

Blend on high to create a puree. When complete, pour the puree into a large bowl. Drain the liquid from the cut cabbage and combine the puree with the cabbage. Add the red pepper flakes. Mix well by hand. Let the kimchi ferment in a sealed container in your fridge. Try a little each day to see how much fermenting you prefer taste wise.

– **Probiotics and immunity:** A healthy gut is also critical to a healthy immune system. In fact, 70–80 percent of our immune tissue is located in the digestive system!

It also seems that a healthy gut seems to regulate levels of the body's main antioxidant, glutathione, which fights a host of diseases.[68]

Experts also indicate that people with certain diseases often have a very different mix of bacteria in their intestines compared to healthier people.[69] Some bacteria can help strengthen the immune system[70] and even prevent obesity,[71] while others can promote inflammation. And what's more, it's not one particular type of bacteria that makes a difference; it's a diversity of bacteria that's turning out to create a more healthful balance in the body.[72]

In fact, a lack of diversity in the diet—so common in a typical American diet rich in processed foods but not in a diverse Mediterranean diet—results in a lack of diversity of gut microbes. Some researchers believe this loss of dietary diversity might be a contributing factor to obesity, type 2 diabetes, gastrointestinal issues, and other health problems.[73]

The Benefits of Fermented Foods

Cultures worldwide have been taking in healthy bacteria—or living organisms—for hundreds if not thousands of years, typically through fermented local foods. (Fermentation helped preserve foods years ago, but many local cultures have also made the link between these fermented foods and better health.) Here's a sampling of some of the indigenous foods different cultures ate (and, in some cases, still eat today):

– During the Roman era, people consumed sauerkraut (cabbage fermented with salt).

– In ancient India, it was common to enjoy lassi, a predinner sour-milk-based yogurt drink that's rich in healthy bacteria.

– In Bulgaria, people regularly drank fermented milk and kefir (also popular today).

– Ukrainians consumed healthy bacteria from raw yogurt, sauerkraut, and buttermilk (a fermented dairy product).

– Asian cultures regularly ate (and eat today) pickled fermentations of cabbage, turnips, eggplant, cucumbers, onions, squash, and carrots.

All these foods are rich in local microorganisms that help balance the gut.

Some studies even show that eating fermented foods like sauerkraut helps prevent disease. Researchers have found that the fermentation process increases the availability of key nutrients (like the cancer-fighting compound sulforaphane), making sauerkraut even healthier than the cabbage from which it was created. In studies of Polish women, researchers found that those who ate lots of sauerkraut had lower rates of breast cancer than those who didn't eat it (or ate much less of it).[74]

Importance of local foods. Some experts are saying that local foods contain a diverse community of *local* microorganisms that are good for your particular digestion—and your gut overall—helping reduce gas and bloating and increasing regularity. The theory: each region has certain bacteria indigenous to that region and to the people in that region that can help those people stay healthy.

This idea of a healthy gut goes way beyond probiotics, which are healthy bacteria or live microorganisms like *Lactobacillus*, *Streptococcus thermophilus,* and *Bifidobacterium* that are often found in yogurt, kefir, some types of cheeses, and many supplements. These probiotics have helped many people regulate their digestive system by creating a better balance of healthy bacteria in the gut (also called "intestinal flora").

The healthy skin/probiotics link. The health of our skin also reflects this internal environment of our gut—as well as the balance of bacteria on our skin. We're quick to blame bacteria for causing problems like acne, but what many don't realize is we need a healthy balance of bacteria on the skin, too, for healthy, problem-free skin.

Skin disorders such as acne rosacea, psoriasis, and dermatitis have been linked with gut problems (including food allergies and leaky-gut syndrome). This may be why research shows that probiotics may help treat atopic dermatitis,[75] a type of eczema where the skin is super sensitive, dry, scaly, and itchy.

Detoxification and Cleansing: The Truth

We hear so much about miracle "detox" cleansing regimens—from juice cleanses to sweat lodges. These are all based on the concept that we need to rid our bodies of toxins (from food, stress, and environmental pollutants) to get back into "balance". The truth is: our bodies have an efficient way of processing toxins through our liver, kidneys, gastrointestinal tract, and skin (through sweat). I believe the best way to "cleanse" is to maintain good health on a daily basis. A few "detoxing" rules:

✓ **Don't smoke** or spend time in the presence of cigarette or cigar smoke.

✓ **Limit alcohol**. An occasional glass of red wine, which is part of the Mediterranean style of eating, is okay.

✓ **Eat organic produce**, limiting your exposure to pesticides.

✓ **Limit your use of plastics**, which contain chemical toxins like BPA.

✓ **Eat a diet rich in fruits, vegetables and whole grains** and low in processed foods, which naturally support the body's ability to detox.

✓ **Whenever possible, drink purified water** (use a water filter to filter out known chemicals like chlorine, lead, and arsenic).

✓ **Use natural-based cleaning products and personal care products**, which limit your exposure to potential toxins.

✓ **Exercise regularly**, which forces the body to sweat and naturally release toxins.

✓ **Practice stress management**; this allows the body to achieve a state of calm.

✓ **Get enough of the detox nutrient, selenium.** Selenium is an essential trace mineral found in protein-rich foods like seafood and nuts. (It's also found in red meat, though I recommend eating this infrequently.)

The right balance of bacteria *on* the skin, too, contributes to the defense mechanisms of the skin (aka proper immune-system functioning). That's why an imbalance on the skin—as in the gut—can contribute to conditions like atopic dermatitis.[76]

There's definitely something to this idea that bacteria—particularly local bacteria from the areas in which we live—is helpful to our health! So if you need even more reason to eat local, or to add fermented foods to your daily diet, this is just another compelling reason.

Step-by-Step Beyond Beauty Diet

The core principles of eating, below, incorporate the Mediterranean style of eating that I've already discussed, as well as my own core beliefs when it comes to holistic health. This, I wholeheartedly believe, is where true inner and outer beauty begins.

~ BEYOND BEAUTY RECIPE ~
Mediterranean Stuffed Tomatoes

This is one of my all-time favorite tomato dishes because it's super easy. You just cook the pasta and then mix these ingredients—or get creative with your own mix-ins. Then bake. These stuffed tomatoes are chockfull of antioxidants and vitamin C—all important for healthy, radiant skin and a healthy body.

Ingredients
1 package whole-wheat orzo pasta
1 small handful organic parsley, chopped
3 ounces organic feta cheese, crumbled
1 small handful organic mint leaves, chopped
1 organic cucumber, diced
¼ cup pine nuts, toasted
2 Tablespoons organic extra virgin olive oil
1 teaspoon organic lemon juice
6 organic tomatoes, tops cut off and cored
Organic salad greens (optional)
* *You can also add grass-fed ground beef to this if you want.*

Directions
Cook pasta, drain, and add rest of ingredients to taste. Place inside fresh, whole organic tomatoes. Bake the tomatoes for 30 minutes at 350°F. Serve warm with salad greens.

Step One

Eat locally grown, organic fruits and vegetables whenever possible. For food to be certified organic, it has to meet guidelines set by the United States Department of Agriculture (USDA). It means fruits and vegetables have to be grown without the use of conventional pesticides or fertilizers made with synthetic ingredients. It also means produce can't be bioengineered or grown with ionizing radiation.

There's been (and continues to be) so much debate over whether or not organic foods are more nutritious, but I stand firmly in the camp that they *are* more nutritious—and just plain better for you. Just look at the diet of the Okinawans and the Ikarians; they were eating locally grown (from their own gardens) fruits and vegetables—not produce grown with pesticides.

Higher in nutrients: One study, in the *Journal of Applied Nutrition*, was conducted over the course of two years.[77] It found that, when compared to conventional foods, organic foods averaged:

- ✓ 63 percent higher in calcium
- ✓ 78 percent higher in chromium
- ✓ 73 percent higher in iron
- ✓ 118 percent higher in magnesium
- ✓ 178 percent higher in molybdenum
- ✓ 91 percent higher in phosphorus
- ✓ 125 percent higher in potassium
- ✓ 60 percent higher in zinc

All of these are key nutrients needed by the body—and the skin. And many of these nutrients are found in the peel (where pesticides can also become concentrated).

In particular, the color of a fruit or vegetable is concentrated in the peel; this colorful part can be a concentrated source of antioxidants called phytochemicals. Tomatoes, for example, have 98 percent of their flavonols (powerful phytochemicals or antioxidants) in their skins. And in the case of potatoes, the skin has more antioxidants, iron, potassium, B vitamins, and fiber than the flesh. The peels are also good sources of something called insoluble fiber, which helps keep you regular. Some peels (like that of an apple) are also rich in soluble fiber that's been shown to help lower cholesterol and control blood sugar.[78]

I've found that the "Dirty Dozen" list published by the Environmental Working Group—a nonprofit organization dedicated to protecting health and the environment—is extremely helpful.[79] This lists the fruits and vegetables that have the top amounts of pesticide residue on their skin (meaning you should eat these foods—out of all others—organic). Topping this list: apples, strawberries, grapes, and celery.

Also something to consider: organic fruits and vegetables use natural waxes on their skins—instead of petroleum-based waxes—that are made from carnauba wax (from the carnauba palm tree) and beeswax.

Conventional fruits and vegetables are also often treated with fungicides, bactericides, and growth regulators—and sometimes even dyed to enhance the color.[80] Organic foods don't use these, which may be why they may sometimes look a little less appealing at the grocery store.

Lower in mercury: When compared to conventionally raised food, organically raised food averaged 29 percent lower in mercury—an environmental toxin that's been linked to neurological problems, particularly in infants and children, and even cancer.[81]

Better for your brain: Research also shows that some commonly used pesticides may alter the development of the brain's dopamine system—responsible for emotional expression and cognitive function—and increase the risk of attention deficit/hyperactivity disorder (ADHD) in children.[82] This effect, researchers found, may persist through adulthood.

Despite the fact that a recent, highly publicized Stanford University review, published in the *Annals of Internal Medicine*, found that organic produce contains no more nutrients than conventional produce—contradicting the earlier study described above—it did find that organic food contained less pesticide residue than conventionally grown foods.[83]

Don't trigger inflammation: I firmly agree that pesticides—no matter what the amount—are not good for your body or for your skin; they trigger the production of something called free radicals in the body, as well as triggering inflammation, which we've already discussed is a precursor to disease.

How can pesticides trigger inflammation? Chemicals in our environment like pesticides and insecticides—used on our food supply and in home gardens—have a strong estrogenic effect on our bodies. Too much exposure to these chemicals can trigger inflammation in the body and may be linked to diseases like breast cancer.[84]

And if these aren't enough reasons to reach for organic fruits and vegetables, at least look for locally grown produce (many farms don't have enough money to get a USDA organic certification but don't use pesticides on their produce, so you should always ask). Many nutrients, particularly heat- and light-sensitive vitamins B and C, are lost in the shipping process, as are fat-soluble nutrients like vitamins A and E and carotenoids (including lycopene).[85]

In one study, conducted at Penn State University, researchers found that the nutrient content of spinach—particularly its folate (vitamin B_9) and carotenoid content—gets quickly lost the longer it's stored.[86] The faster fresh food makes it to your table (the idea behind the popular food-to-table movement) and the fewer pesticides it contains, the more nutritious that food will be for you.

There is one exception: frozen fruits and vegetables. These foods are picked at the height of their freshness and undergo a process called flash freezing (often done right where they're picked), allowing them to avoid the loss of nutrients from shipping and storage. In fact, some studies have found that frozen fruits and vegetables are just as nutritious as fresh.[87] One particular study was done by researchers at South Dakota State University;[88] it found that the antioxidant content of blueberries was maintained when frozen. And, what's more, the researchers found that freezing actually improves the availability of the antioxidants in the body.

Why Free Radicals Trigger Disease

You'll hear me talking a lot about free radicals throughout this book. Here's a little Science 101 about what they are—and why they're not always good for your body, your health, or your skin.

Our bodies are made up of different kinds of cells. These cells are made up of different kinds of molecules. And these molecules are made up of atoms. Free radicals are atoms or groups of atoms with an unpaired or odd number of negatively charged particles called electrons. Electrons typically come in pairs, which makes these unpaired electrons—also called free radicals—highly unstable, or reactive.

They attack cells in the body in an effort to steal an electron to become stable again; in the process, the molecule with the stolen electron becomes a free radical. This chain reaction occurs unless stopped by antioxidants, which donate an electron to the free radicals, thus stabilizing them.[89]

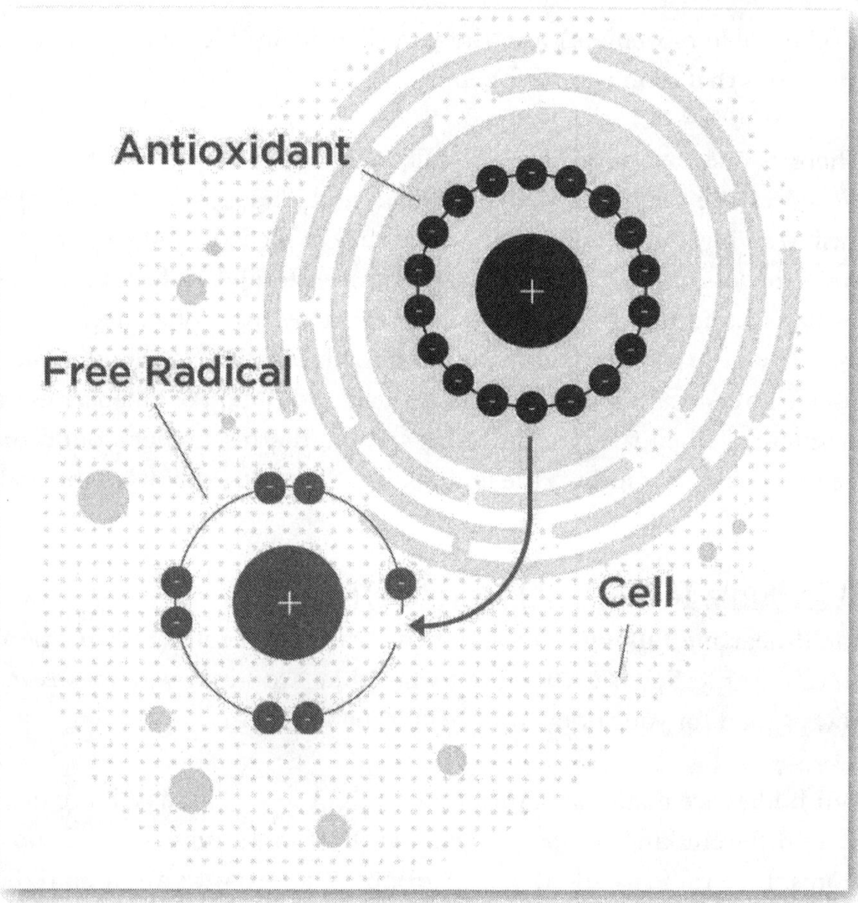

When a molecule loses an electron, it becomes a highly unstable free radical—which can trigger health problems and premature aging. Antioxidants neutralize or stabilize free radical molecules by donating an electron to them.

These attacks by free radicals change the structure and function of cells and how they work, disrupting the cell and often its DNA and RNA. Cellular damage caused by free radicals is a key part of the aging process—and may even contribute to the development of some of our most prevalent diseases, including cancer.[90]

There are five major free radicals found in the skin: hydroxyl, peroxyl, peroxynitrite, singlet oxygen, and superoxide anion.[91] These can break down collagen and elastin, as well as lipids in the skin, triggering premature aging (think wrinkles, sagging skin, and hyperpigmentation or brown spots) and even contributing to skin cancer.

How do free radicals develop in the first place? Sometimes, free radicals develop as a byproduct from our body's own processes like cellular metabolism and from digestion (particularly when we eat highly processed or fried foods). They can also be created as a result of exercise. (When cells use oxygen to generate energy, free radicals are created.[92]) They can also develop from exposure to pollutants—air pollution and car exhaust, cigarette smoke, pesticides in our environment and in our food—as well as from the sun's ultraviolet radiation.[93]

Step Two

Eat less red meat. I love a good barbecue every once in a while, but red meat should be limited, if possible, to less than four times a month. Research has found that the more red meat you eat, the higher your markers of inflammation.[94]

Consumption of red meat has also been linked to breast cancer. Research done in countries with low red-meat consumption found there to be a lower incidence of breast cancer.[95] As Western fast-food diets have become more popular in these countries, breast-cancer numbers have risen—particularly in women who eat more red meat. Other research from Harvard University found that weekly red-meat consumption of about eighteen ounces or more (a serving size is about three ounces, though many people in America easily eat an eight-ounce steak) raises breast cancer risk.[96] Red meat has also been shown to worsen kidney disease—which affects twenty-six million people in the United States. People with chronic kidney disease who consume diets high in protein like red meat are three times more likely to develop kidney failure than patients who consume diets high in fruits in vegetables.[97]

If you're going to eat red meat once in a while, opt for grass-fed red meat. Conventionally raised red meat contains too-high levels of unhealthy omega-6 fatty acids. Organic grass-fed red meat is rich in inflammation-quelling omega-3 fatty acids.

~ BEYOND BEAUTY RECIPE ~
Portobello Burgers

Portobello mushrooms are a good source of fiber and B vitamins, as well as the antioxidant minerals selenium and potassium. The B vitamins help boost circulation in the body—including in the skin, which can help give you a healthy, radiant glow.

Ingredients
3 organic Portobello mushrooms
4 Tablespoons balsamic vinegar
¼ cup organic extra virgin olive oil
Pinch pink Himalayan sea salt
Pinch pepper
¼ cup organic lemon juice
4 organic garlic cloves, crushed
1 organic onion, sliced (optional)
Organic feta cheese (optional)

Directions
Clean mushrooms and remove stems. Combine the remaining ingredients in a bowl, and marinate the mushrooms for 3 hours. Then grill to desired doneness (about 10 minutes) and top with grilled sliced organic onion and organic feta cheese.

Don't char your meat. When you do eat meat—be it red meat or lean meat like poultry—don't char it. These grill marks and crispy bits on hamburgers, steaks, or other meat are laden with carcinogenic compounds called AGEs or advanced glycation end products. (The more char, the more AGEs.) AGEs promote inflammation by damaging essential proteins in the body and turning them into inflammatory agents harmful to cells. Numerous studies have linked AGEs with an increased risk of cancer,[98] Alzheimer's disease, and diabetes.[99]

If you have to grill, precook meat over low heat in a skillet or oven first to reduce the amount of time needed to cook at higher heat. Better cooking methods altogether include baking, poaching, stewing, and steaming. Using rosemary (an herb super high in health-promoting antioxidants) on your meat—before grilling it—can also help reduce the formation of unhealthy AGEs, according to one study.[100] Another study found that soaking meat in a vinegar- or citrus-based marinade, along with antioxidant-rich herbs like rosemary, also helps reduce the formation of AGEs.[101]

Step Three

Incorporate olive oil into your daily diet. Extra-virgin olive oil is a staple of the Mediterranean style of eating. Not only is olive oil delicious, but it's superhealthy for you, too, because it contains very high levels of monounsaturated fats (particularly oleic acid) that studies suggest may be linked to a reduced risk of heart disease.[102] Because extra-virgin olive oil is the first extract from the olives, it's typically cold pressed (make sure it says this on the label) and not heat processed. This allows for a higher concentration of antioxidants.

~ BEYOND BEAUTY RECIPE ~
Black Olive Crusted Haddock

Fish is rich in omega-3 fatty acids, which are good for your body, as well as for your skin and hair. You can substitute your favorite fish in place of haddock, if you want. Just make sure it's one that's low in mercury—a neurotoxin that's been linked to a host of health problems including neurological disorders. Other low-mercury seafood includes tilapia, flounder, perch, sole, salmon, sardines, scallops, and shrimp.

Ingredients
1 cup oil-cured black olives*
2 cups breadcrumbs
2 cloves organic garlic
1 organic shallot
½ bunch organic parsley
½ bunch organic chives
Organic grapeseed oil (for searing)
Organic extra virgin olive oil, as needed

Directions
Combine olives, breadcrumbs, garlic, shallots, and herbs in a food processor, and pulse until olives are chopped and breadcrumbs are softened. Drizzle in extra olive oil to soften breadcrumbs. Drizzle grapeseed oil (which can be used at very high heat) in the pan, heat pan, then place fish on it and sear just one side. (Searing adds caramelized texture to the outside of the fish, while leaving the inside flaky and tender.) Turn fish over, place in a glass dish and top with olive oil and breadcrumb mixture. Bake the haddock in a 350°F oven for 20 minutes.

Rich in antioxidants: There's evidence that the antioxidants in olive oil—simple phenols, secoiridoids, lignans, oleic acid (also called omega-9), and squalene[103]—improve cholesterol regulation and LDL cholesterol reduction.[104] Squalene is also known for its skin-health benefits. Olive oil can help repair skin damage; soothe and relieve chapped, itchy skin; and help rebuild skin's moisture barrier, which keeps skin hydrated.

It's no surprise, then, that researchers, in the journal *Burn,* found that when burn patients consumed olive oil, their wounds healed faster than those of patients who didn't consume olive oil.[105] The reason, researchers theorized: olive oil has significant anti-inflammatory and antioxidant benefits, which help optimize wound healing.

Just to show you how powerful a health food olive oil is: another study found that adding as little as ten teaspoons of olive oil to your daily diet could help protect women against breast cancer. The Spanish researchers theorize that olive oil may mount a multipronged attack on cancer tumors, stunting their growth, and even protect against potentially cancerous damage to DNA.[106]

What's more, compelling research found that olecanthal—a powerful antioxidant found in extra-virgin olive oil—has been shown to wipe out cancer cells in as little as thirty minutes.[107] This is the kind of science that's so impressive it's hard not to sit up and take notice—or at least revamp your diet to be more like the Okinawans or the Ikarians!

Choosing the right olive oil: Look for olive oils that come in a dark bottle, which protects against light. Exposure to light can cause the oil to deteriorate. Also, steer clear of giant tins: olive oils are best used within three to six months. To keep it fresh, store your oil in a cool, dark place.

Step Four

Store food in glass containers, and avoid eating or drinking from plastic containers. Avoid buying your milk or juice in those plastic jugs. And be careful, too, of what kind of canned goods you buy; many have a plastic lining, which contains the chemical BPA—bisphenol A—on the inside. Just as pesticides can have estrogenic effects in the body that can affect your health, so too can plastics[108]—which contain chemicals like PVC[109] (or polyvinyl chloride), BPA, and phthalates that have been linked to health problems like cancer.

One study, published in the *Journal of Clinical Endocrinology & Metabolism*, found that men, women, and children exposed to high levels of phthalates (chemicals found in plastics—even in plastic baby teethers[110]—and some personal-care products) tend to have reduced levels of testosterone in their blood compared to those with lower chemical exposure.[111] While testosterone is the main sex hormone in men, it contributes to a variety of functions in both men and women, including physical growth and strength, brain function, bone density, and cardiovascular health.

Another study found that extensive exposure to common chemicals found in plastics is linked to an earlier start of menopause in women.[112]

Additional research shows that even low levels of exposure to phthalates by mothers who were pregnant affected male infants' reproductive health later in life.[113] As more scientific research points to the negative health consequences of exposure to chemicals in plastics, I become more convinced about limiting our exposure.

This brings up the question on how to limit our exposure. Here are some helpful tips from the National Institutes of Health[114] and other experts when it comes to plastics:

✓ **Don't microwave polycarbonate plastic food containers.** Plastic is a synthetic material made up of a group of substances called polymers. And while polycarbonate—one type of plastic—seems strong and durable (and almost glass like), it may break down from overuse at high temperatures. A breakdown in plastics causes chemicals in the plastics to potentially leach into food or drink. A good rule of thumb to follow is to never microwave any kind of plastic—polycarbonate, plastic wrap, or any other kind. I would also argue, for this same reason, not to put plastics in the dishwasher; hand wash them to be safe. If you must put them in the dishwasher, only put them on the top rack. The bottom rack is near the heating element, which can cause the plastic to heat up even more.

✓ **Know that BPA free doesn't mean chemical free.** BPA is an industrial chemical used primarily to make hard polycarbonate plastic and other types of plastics (it's the chemical that hardens plastics). It's found in dental sealants, water bottles, the lining of canned foods and drinks, and many other products.

The problem with this chemical is that it's an endocrine disruptor—a chemical that mimics hormones like estrogen—triggering oxidative damage[115] and long-term health problems like cancer,[116] as well as other serious brain and behavioral problems (including autism[117]), particularly in pregnant women, children, and infants. It's also been linked to higher blood pressure.[118]

And just because something has been labeled BPA free doesn't mean that it doesn't contain other potentially harmful chemicals. Many of the replacements for BPA have not been thoroughly tested for their effects on your health.[119] More studies need to be done. Chemicals of any kind can leach into food or drinks, particularly if the plastic gets heated up.

In one particularly concerning University of Florida study, published in the journal *Environmental Pollution*, it was found that when plastic water bottles (the kind you buy from a store to drink on the go) were left in the heat of a car for weeks, the water had increased levels of the chemicals antimony (considered a carcinogen by the International Agency for

Research on Cancer) and BPA—which leached into the drinking water from the plastic.[120]

✓ **When possible, opt for glass, porcelain, or stainless-steel containers**, particularly for hot food or liquids—especially your water bottle that you drink from every day.

Step Five

Reduce your use of canned foods. My philosophy when it comes to food: fresh is always best. When you can't use fresh, frozen is the next best option. Canned food is typically high in sodium and low in nutrients, which is why I try to avoid it. The only exception to this rule is canned beans, which are precooked. And if you check the labels, you can find ones that contain low to no sodium.

High in sodium: Did you know that just one teaspoon of salt contains 2,300 milligrams (mg) of sodium, but your body only needs 200 mg of sodium per day? That's a big discrepancy! In fact, the average American takes in anywhere from 3,000 to 3,600 mg of sodium daily.[121]

You need a proper balance of sodium (e.g., table salt, which is sodium chloride) and water in the body in order to function properly. If you eat too many salty or processed foods (which sneak in a lot of sodium), you can upset this equilibrium, causing the body to hold on to water. This puts an extra burden on your heart or blood vessels, often triggering high blood pressure. It can also make your eyes and face look puffy.

~ BEYOND BEAUTY RECIPE ~
3-Bean Super Salad

Beans are chockfull of nutrients like protein and fiber—and are a perfect replacement in your diet for red meat. This is one of my favorite bean recipes that I make for my family (and one that my grandmother and mother made for me, too, years ago).

Ingredients
15 oz cannellini (white kidney) beans
15 oz garbanzo beans
15 oz red kidney beans
½ organic onion, minced
1 clove organic garlic, minced
2 tablespoons minced fresh, organic parsley
¼ cup organic, extra virgin olive oil
1 organic lemon, juiced
Salt and black pepper, to taste
1 large organic tomato, chopped (optional)

Directions
Combine cannellini, garbanzo, and red kidney beans in a mixing bowl. Add onion, garlic, parsley, olive oil, lemon juice, salt, pepper, and tomato. Mix well with a spoon. Serve as a side dish or as a main course over organic mixed greens.

A Mediterranean diet, which focuses on fresh, healthy, unprocessed food, is naturally low in sodium. So is the DASH diet (Dietary Approaches to Stop Hypertension). This diet borrows many of the healthy-eating principles of the Mediterranean diet (eating fresh fruits and vegetables, unrefined grains, nuts and seeds, legumes, lean protein, and healthy fats) but also focuses on reducing sodium overall by limiting the amount of processed foods you're eating and the amount of table salt you're added to foods.

Studies show that by following the DASH diet, you may be able to reduce your blood pressure by a few points in just two weeks—and your systolic blood pressure (which results from your heart muscle contracting) could drop by seven to twelve points over time.[122] This could make a significant difference in your long-term health.

High in BPA: One other concern I have with canned foods is not only the sodium and nutrient levels, but also the BPA that's used to create the inner linings of cans. This toxic chemical can and does leach into canned foods like beans. When shopping, look for canned foods that are BPA free. I've also found that organic canned foods are typically manufactured without any additional chemicals like BPA that could cause potential health problems.

High in aluminum: Another toxin to consider is aluminum. Used to manufacture most cans, foil, and juice pouches, aluminum is a neurotoxin. Exposure to it has been implicated in a number of neurological diseases including Alzheimer's.[123] Does that mean you should never eat anything from a can, wrap anything in aluminum foil, or let your child drink out of a juice pouch? No, it just means that you should limit your exposure and your family's exposure whenever it makes sense.

Step Six

Steer clear of genetically modified foods or GMOs. My belief: the closer you get to the most natural form of a fruit or vegetable—without any sort of man-made manipulation, be it genetic modifications or pesticides—the better for your health. That's why I'm not a fan of GMO foods.

There is some concern that these foods might contain lower amounts of nutrients, particularly phytoestrogens[124]—potent antioxidants that have been linked to lower rates of cancers and heart disease.[125]

And there have been some concerning studies linking GMO foods to serious diseases like cancer. One study, by scientist Judy Carman, published in the peer-reviewed *Journal of Organic Systems,* showed the effects of a diet of mixed GMO feed for pigs. It caused some disturbing health problems, particularly regarding the pigs' digestive, reproductive, and endocrine systems.[126] This study has been widely criticized by the GMO industry, but in my opinion, the results of this study are too concerning to ignore. Until we know exactly how GMO foods affect our health, my advice is to avoid them whenever you can.

Step Seven

Eat seasonally. Eating foods when nature produces them (the concept of eating seasonally) is something the Mediterranean culture and people all over the world have done throughout history. At its very core, seasonal eating is local eating. It means building your meals around foods that have been harvested at their peak on local farms, and it means modifying your diet according to the season.

When the food you're eating isn't in season (e.g., you're eating watermelon in winter), it's either been grown in a greenhouse or shipped in from other parts of the world—both of which affect taste and nutrient content. When transporting crops, they must be harvested early and refrigerated so they don't rot during transportation. They may not ripen as effectively as they would in their natural environment, and as a result they don't develop their full flavor. In addition, transporting produce sometimes requires irradiation (zapping the produce with a burst of radiation to kill germs) and preservatives (such as petroleum-based wax) to protect the produce and increase shelf life.

~ BEYOND BEAUTY RECIPE ~
Stuffed Grape Leaves

Grape leaves are a staple of the Mediterranean region—and are rich in fiber, and vitamins A and K, as well as calcium and iron. These stuffed grape leaves have been passed down from my mother's side of the family. They make a perfect appetizer or main course, when served with a side of vegetables.

Ingredients
1 16-ounce jar grape leaves
1 pound lean ground grass-fed beef*
2 cups organic rice
2 organic eggs
½ chopped organic onion
½ cup extra virgin olive oil
½ cup organic lemon juice
1 clove organic garlic, crushed
2 pounds organic tomatoes, diced
Pinch, pink Himalayan sea salt
Pinch, ground black pepper
1 Tablespoon, fresh organic chopped mint (optional)
1 Tablespoon, fresh organic chopped parsley (optional)

Directions
Mix together all ingredients except grape leaves. (You can also mix in the fresh chopped mint and/or parsley if you want.) Place mixture inside grape leaves and roll to close. Place on top of each other in a large pot and fill ¾ of the way with water. Add olive oil and lemon juice. Boil over medium heat until tender, and desired doneness (about 45 minutes).

** If you're going to eat red meat, grass-fed red meat is the healthiest choice because it's been shown to trigger less inflammation in the body (it contains less pro-inflammatory omega-6 fatty acids and more anti-inflammatory omega-3 fatty acids).*

Many cultures, including Indian culture and its ancient medicine called ayurveda, believe that nature harvests the antidotes for the season. For example, warming and nourishing foods like root vegetables, soups and stews, and fermented foods like tempeh and kimchi help build protein and fat reserves in the body for the long winter season ahead. According to ayurvedic expert John Douillard, our digestive fires have evolved to be stronger in winter, allowing us to eat more dense foods than we would in summer.[127] And in summer, our fires are weaker, which allows us to eat less-dense foods like salads and fresh berries.

Step Eight

Eat fish, which are rich in omega-3 fatty acids. These healthy fats—also called essential fatty acids—are found in everything from wild-caught salmon, sardines, and tilapia to flaxseeds, chia seeds, and walnuts. Studies have shown that these fats can do everything from boosting your mood[128] to protecting cognitive function[129] and preventing Alzheimer's disease.[130]

One reason they have such a health-promoting effect is that they decrease inflammation. They also seem to reduce oxidative stress and cell death, which can lead to diseases like cancer.

In one 2013 review of twenty-one studies, Chinese researchers found that women with the highest intake of omega-3 fatty acids from seafood had a 14 percent lower risk of breast cancer. In fact, just a miniscule increase in omega-3-rich seafood every day (about 0.004 ounces) was associated with a 5 percent lower risk of breast cancer.

Rich in vitamin B_3: Fish (tuna, sardines, and wild salmon)—as well as mushrooms, asparagus, tomatoes, peanuts, bell peppers, sweet potatoes, sunflower seeds, and brown rice—are all high in vitamin B_3 (also called niacin or nicotinaminde). One study found that this vitamin can significantly reduce rates of nonmelanoma skin cancers in patients.[131]

This critical vitamin is a potent antioxidant that helps quench free radicals (created by exposure to sunlight, among other things) and protect against excessive tissue damage. In fact, the Australian researchers who conducted the study theorize that vitamin B_3 may enhance DNA repair in skin cells damaged by sunlight and offer protection against the sun's ultraviolet light. (Sunscreen is still essential, though; this nutrient just offers additional protection against cancer.)

If you're not getting enough of this nutrient from the foods you eat, talk to your doctor about taking a supplement. Though researchers studied this water-soluble vitamin using twice-daily doses of 500 mg, the RDA (recommended daily allowance) of vitamin B_3 is 14 mg for women and 16 mg for men. However, if you're deficient or have skin cancer, you may need more.

Step Nine

Add more color to your diet. The more colorful the food, the higher the content of health-promoting antioxidants. Some of my favorite colorful, antioxidant-rich foods include berries (acai berries, blueberries, raspberries, strawberries, and blackberries), citrus fruits like red grapefruit and oranges, pomegranates, and grapes.

Here's a guide to what colorful fruits and vegetables can offer you and your health:

- **Green** Veggies like kale, spinach, purslane (similar to watercress and spinach), and broccoli are high in lutein, which helps keep your vision sharp. (The same holds true for the Asian favorites: kombu, or edible kelp; hijiki, which is common in seaweed salads; and wakame, or edible seaweed.) They're also high in the antioxidant vitamin C, which is critical for healthy, youthful-looking skin—and the production of collagen, the tissue-firming protein that acts as a scaffold for the skin.

- **Yellow/orange** Mangoes, carrots, sweet potatoes, and pumpkin all contain antioxidants called carotenoids that can reduce the risk of developing cancer. They can also give your complexion a healthy glow—so often used to characterize youthful skin.[132]

~ BEYOND BEAUTY RECIPE ~
Garlic-y Kale

Kale is an amazing source of nutrients like vitamins A, C, and K and minerals like manganese, copper, and iron. It's great for the skin—and the body. (Not to mention, it contains olive oil and garlic, both of which are super healthy for you, too.) Here's one of the recipes I frequently make with my family; it's quick and so good for you!

Ingredients
1 bunch organic kale
2 tablespoons organic, extra virgin olive oil
1 clove organic garlic, minced
1 small organic onion, minced (optional)
1 large organic tomato, chopped (optional)
Salt and pepper, to taste
Red pepper flakes, to taste (optional)

Directions
Remove kale leaves from the stems; rinse under cool water. Heat 2 tablespoons of olive oil and 1 clove minced garlic in a large skillet over medium heat. Once the oil is hot, add the washed kale to the skillet and cover. Stir occasionally, and continue to cook until the kale is wilted. (To add variety, add 1 small onion, minced and sautéed and/or 1 large chopped tomato.) Don't overcook. Season with salt and pepper and/or red pepper flakes to taste.

• **Blue/purple** Berries like blueberries, acai berries, and blackberries—as well as purple potatoes and purple cauliflower—are chock-full of antioxidant-rich substances called anthocyanins. These can help prevent tumors from forming, including tumors on the skin, and may even suppress their growth.[133]

• **Red** Watermelon and tomatoes are rich in lycopene (a carotenoid), which may protect against cancer[134] and heart disease and boosts your skin's radiance. And when it comes to the skin, lycopene also has a natural UV-protective capability.[135] The reason may be that lyocopene is a scavenger of free radicals, which are created when the skin is exposed to the sun. But this doesn't mean you don't need sunscreen. This natural sun protection is just another reason that eating healthy—including colorful fruits and vegetables—can slow down the aging process of the skin, particularly when exposed to the damaging effects of the sun's ultraviolet rays.

Step Ten

Eat dark chocolate—in moderation. White sugar may increase inflammation and reduce immunity, but that doesn't mean you should forgo sweets altogether. In fact, dark chocolate (with at least 70 percent cocoa content) is one of the healthiest sweets you can indulge in—in moderation (remember: it's still high in calories). The reason: it's chock-full of substances called flavonoids, and specifically flavonoids called procyanidins and epicatechins. Flavonoids are part of a group of antioxidants known as polyphenols (the same antioxidants found in red wine, green tea, and grapes). Dark chocolate also contains minerals like calcium, magnesium, and potassium, which are good for the body and for the skin.

Good for the heart: But it's what dark chocolate seems to do for the heart that makes it such a health-promoting food. In one study, scientists found that dark chocolate helps restore flexibility to the arteries while also preventing white blood cells from sticking to the walls of blood vessels.[136] (Both arterial stiffness and this white blood cell "adhesion," as it's called, are known factors that play a significant role in heart disease.)

Good for the skin: Dark chocolate has also shown benefits for the skin, thanks to these high levels of flavonoids. In one study, published in *The*

Journal of Nutrition, German researchers found that eating dark chocolate—specifically one half cup of dark-chocolate cocoa daily—resulted, after just one month, in skin that was smoother, more hydrated, and less scaly and red when exposed to ultraviolet light.[137] The researchers speculated that the flavonoids help absorb UV light, protecting the skin and increasing blood flow and hydration.

~ BEYOND BEAUTY RECIPE ~
Organic Zucchini with Fresh Herbs

Zucchini is chockfull of skin-friendly and health-boosting antioxidants like vitamin C, lutein, and zeaxanthin. This is one of my favorite recipes to whip up at home; it's fast, easy, and my kids love it!

Ingredients
8 small organic zucchini (2 lb)
1 teaspoon pink Himalayan sea salt
Dash pepper
¼ cup organic extra virgin olive oil
2 Tablespoons chopped organic parsley
1 Tablespoon snipped organic chives or dill
1 Tablespoon juice from an organic lemon

Directions
Wash zucchini, cut into diagonal, ¼-inch thick slices. In a medium skillet bring ½ cup water with salt and pepper to boil. Add zucchini; cook over medium heat, covered 10 minutes or until just tender. Add olive oil, parsley, chives and lemon juice; toss gently to combine. Pour into serving dish; serve warm.

Step Eleven

Cook with fresh herbs. All herbs—like sage, thyme, peppermint, and lemon balm—are rich in antioxidants that can help fight inflammation. Many herbs, like oregano, are also antimicrobial. In fact, oregano contains an active agent called rosmarinic acid that's superhigh in free-radical-fighting antioxidants.

My favorite herbs are basil, cilantro, dill, ginger, mint, oregano, parsley, rosemary, thyme, cinnamon, garlic, and turmeric. Use them when you're cooking—or just sprinkle them on anything you can—to add flavor and antioxidants.

Benefits of turmeric and curcumin: Curcumin is the most active part of the herb turmeric, which is responsible for the yellow color of Indian curry and American mustard. It's packed with anti-inflammatory and antioxidant properties and has been shown to have numerous benefits, namely:[138]

✓ **It boosts skin health.** As a potent anti-inflammatory, it makes sense that curcumin can help treat inflammatory skin conditions like psoriasis, skin cancer, and scleroderma (an autoimmune disease where the connective tissue in the body—which connects, supports, and surrounds other tissues and organs—becomes hardened and rigid).[139] Curcumin also seems to help reduce the time it takes to heal a wound. What's more, a Japanese study found that curcumin also seems to help protect the skin from the oxidative damage triggered by exposure to the sun's ultraviolet B radiation.[140]

✓ **It may prevent liver damage.** Curcumin seems to delay liver damage that can eventually lead to cirrhosis.[141]

✓ **It may help reduce your risk of cancer.** Adding certain spices like turmeric to meat prior to cooking can reduce levels of heterocyclic amines—carcinogenic compounds formed when meats are barbecued, boiled, or fried—by up to 40 percent.[142]

✓ **It may help prevent the growth of cancer.** Researchers found that curcumin's anticancer potential "stems from its ability to suppress the proliferation of a wide variety of tumor cells."[143] Curcumin also seems to inhibit the growth of the skin cancer melanoma and slow the spread of breast cancer into the lungs.[144]

✓ **It may help make chemotherapy and radiation more effective.** Pretreatment with curcumin seems to make cancer cells more vulnerable to chemo and radiotherapy.[145]

✓ **It may boost your memory.** Adding just one gram of turmeric (about one-quarter of a teaspoon) to your breakfast can help improve working memory, including planning, problem-solving, and reasoning, for over six hours.[146]

✓ **It may lower your risk of Alzheimer's disease.** Scientists believe that the turmeric found in curries eaten daily in India may help explain the low rate of Alzheimer's disease in that country.[147] Among people aged seventy to seventy-nine, the rate is less than one-quarter that of the United States.

Step Twelve

Drink red wine—in moderation. Red wine is chock-full of good-for-you antioxidants,[148] including a class of antioxidants called polyphenols. The most well-known (and well-researched) polyphenol is resveratrol. This potent antioxidant comes from the skin of grapes used to make wine. (Red and purple grape juices may have some of the same heart-healthy benefits of red wine for this reason.[149])

Resveratrol is an anti-inflammatory that helps prevent damage to blood vessels, reduces low-density lipoprotein (LDL) cholesterol (the "bad" cholesterol), and prevents blood clots. Some research also shows that resveratrol could be linked to a reduced risk of inflammation and blood clotting, both of which can lead to heart disease.[150]

While alcohol, in general, isn't good for you, having a glass of red wine in moderation—something that is just one small part of the Mediterranean diet—can turn out to be healthy.

STEP THIRTEEN

Limit the amount of sugar you eat. Anything that causes a fast spike in blood-sugar levels, like white sugar and white flour (found in many processed foods), triggers an inflammatory response in the body. Eat it on a regular basis, and you're keeping your inflammation levels on overdrive.

Sugar has also been known to impair immune function. One landmark study, published in the *American Journal of Clinical Nutrition*, revealed that consuming one hundred grams (3.5 ounces) of carbohydrates, such as fructose, glucose, sucrose, and honey, inhibited the ability of white blood cells to engulf and destroy harmful microorganisms and particles that were foreign to the body.[151] The function of white blood cells was lowered by as much as 50 percent—and impairment of immune function began less than thirty minutes after sugar ingestion and remained this way for more than five hours.

But don't use chemical sweeteners as a sugar substitute. Some research indicates that these sweeteners are so unnaturally sweet that they desensitize people to the natural sweet taste of fresh foods like fruits. Chemical sweeteners also seem to fool the body—so the body doesn't register that it's consumed sugar, causing us to eat more than we should. In fact, other research indicates that artificial sweeteners could cause weight gain by stimulating the development of new fat cells.[152] While these studies aren't exhaustive of all the studies done on chemical sweeteners, the ones that have shown negative effects are particularly concerning—and are enough reason, in my mind, to steer clear of them.

STEP FOURTEEN

Drink enough water. I can't emphasize enough the importance of drinking plain old water. Water helps the body rid itself of toxins. If you drink enough, it flushes out the kidneys and pulls toxins from the body. If you don't drink enough water, your body can't filter properly. And if you get dehydrated, the organs don't function as well.

Proper hydration makes the skin smoother and "plumper" looking, more hydrated, and more radiant overall. Dehydration can cause fine lines and wrinkles to become more obvious. Researchers at the University of Missouri in Columbia found that having just about two cups of water significantly boosted blood flow throughout the body and skin.[153]

If you dislike the taste of plain water, mix in your own healthy flavoring by adding antioxidant-rich frozen organic berries, cold organic cucumbers, or even a splash of fruit juice.

Step Fifteen

Replace saturated fats. These fats are found in everything from fatty meats (beef, lamb, pork) to butter, cheese, and dairy products made from whole or 2 percent milk. Replace these fats with monounsaturated or polyunsaturated fats (found in olives, olive oil, avocados, flaxseed, walnuts, and fish oil).

Olive oil, in particular, has been found to be healthy for you, hands down. Some of the research suggests that the oleic acid found in olive oil may een help reduce breast-cancer risk.[154] Other numerous studies show that polyunsaturated fats can improve cholesterol levels and lower blood pressure, making them much more heart-healthy than saturated fats.

And while I'm on the topic of fats, I also want to mention that you should eliminate trans fats from your diet by avoiding fast food like french fries and processed foods like cookies and pastries. It's also found in solid shortening and stick margarine. There are simply no studies showing that there are any health benefits of trans fats. In fact, of the studies conducted, one found that women who had the highest levels of trans fats in their blood were twice as likely as women with the lowest levels to develop breast cancer.[155] This doesn't surprise me as trans fats are found in the unhealthiest of foods—and eating the right foods, as I've already mentioned, is critical to staying healthy and avoiding disease.

Step Sixteen

Be sure you're getting enough vitamin D. This essential nutrient (actually a hormone) is getting a lot of attention these days—for good reason. Not only does it play an important role, alongside calcium, in strengthening bones, it's also a powerful antioxidant and potent immune booster.[156]

In fact, research shows that cancer patients who had high levels of vitamin D in their bloodstream prior to treatment survived longer than those with lower levels of the vitamin.[157] Researchers from the Dana-Farber Cancer Institute believe this vitamin can perk up the immune system's vigilance against cancer cells.[158] Vitamin D deficiency has also been linked to depression,[159] as well as prediabetes and diabetes.[160] In fact, one study found that people who have low levels of vitamin D are more likely to have diabetes, regardless of how much they weigh.[161]

Vitamin D has also been found to help heal the skin: a daily dose of D (1,000 IU) seems to help treat seasonal atopic dermatitis[162]—itchy, scaly skin that's common during the winter.

Vitamin D is known as the sun vitamin because the body produces it when exposed to the sun. (Our bodies aren't able to produce vitamin D on their own.) But there are plenty of ways to get your daily D without sun exposure, which puts you at risk of skin cancer (and premature skin aging): eat foods rich in vitamin D like salmon, sardines, dairy, and mushrooms, or check in with your doctor about whether you should take a daily supplement. Adults need anywhere from 400 IU to 800 IU daily. Also important: look for vitamin D_3 (or cholecalciferol) instead of vitamin D_2 (called ergocalciferol) on your supplements. Experts say vitamin D_3 is the most readily absorbed and utilized by the body.

STEP SEVENTEEN

Eat spicy foods. Red-hot chili peppers (also called cayenne peppers) contain an ingredient called capsaicin, which makes the peppers incredibly hot to the taste. This fire and heat in the mouth actually triggers the brain to produce a rush of endorphins (the feel-good chemicals that block pain).

By stimulating endorphin production in response to pain, chili peppers, when eaten and when specially formulated in skin creams, have been shown to help treat all types of pain—from arthritis pain to the pain of itchy, inflamed skin. Capsaicin has also been shown to inhibit inflammation in the body.[163]

What's more, this hot spice has also been shown to lower blood pressure, reduce cholesterol levels, and reduce risk of blood clots—boosting cardiovascular health. (Capsaicin blocks the action of a gene that makes the arteries contract, restricting blood flow to the heart and organs. This blocking action allows more blood to flow through the blood vessels.[164])

So it's no wonder that researchers have determined that eating spicy foods (including foods that contain red-hot chili peppers) can boost longevity.[165] These Harvard Medical School researchers have found that capsaicin has antioxidant, antiobesity, anti-inflammation, and anticancer properties.

A word of warning, though: as health promoting as spicy foods can be, they can still aggravate skin conditions like rosacea, which flare up in response to heat and spices. So if you struggle with rosacea, use caution with spicy foods and capsaicin.

STEP EIGHTEEN

Drink coffee. One staple of a Mediterranean diet: a cup of coffee (or two) every day. I've always loved a cup of coffee in the morning—but I've come to love it even more over the years as more and more research is done about its health benefits. I want to recap some of the most recent studies to date, but first I want to share my own coffee story with you.

I've traveled to places like Mexico, Jamaica, and Central America where I've had the opportunity to visit coffee farms. And what I consistently heard and saw was that coffee pickers had hands that were youthful looking—more youthful than the skin on the rest of their bodies, which was showing all the normal signs of aging (thanks to many hours spent in the sun): weathered, rough skin; wrinkles; and age spots. But the hands—which came into contact daily with the fruit of the coffee plant—were not.

It was then that I discovered that this fruit of the coffee plant (one type of which is called *Coffea arabica*) is one of the richest sources of health-promoting and antiaging antioxidants. *Coffea arabica* is also a superhealthy coffee to drink because it's chock-full of antioxidants. Numerous studies are now backing up the benefits of all coffee:

• **It helps you live longer.** Harvard researchers have found that people who drink three to five cups of coffee a day were 15 percent less likely to die of any cause when compared with people who didn't drink coffee.[166]

• **It lowers your cancer risk.** Research presented at the American Association of Cancer Researchers meeting in San Diego suggests that people who drink at least a cup a day have a lower risk of liver cancer compared to those who only indulge occasionally.[167] Study participants were tracked for eighteen years; it was the regular coffee drinkers who had up to a 42 percent reduced risk of this type of cancer. Beyond liver cancer, studies have suggested that coffee may be tied to a reduced risk of head and neck cancers, colorectal cancers, prostate cancer, and bladder, endometrial,[168] esophageal, and pancreatic cancers. Additional research also shows that coffee (in amounts of just two cups daily) protects against breast-cancer recurrence in women.[169]

Researchers theorize that coffee helps inhibit the growth of tumors by "turning off" signaling pathways that cancer cells require to grow.

• **It protects against melanoma.** This is a dangerous form of skin cancer and can be deadly if not treated. Research from the National Cancer Institute found that drinking four or more cups of coffee per day reduces the risk of malignant melanoma by 20 percent.[170] This is a lot of coffee—so also keep moderation in mind. How I interpret it: drink your regular cup or two each day, and use daily protection of sunscreen (and sun-smart strategies) to help protect against skin cancer.

• **It keeps your heart healthy.** Drinking two eight-ounce cups of coffee each day helps reduce your risk of heart failure by 11 percent, according to a study in the journal *Circulation: Heart Failure*.[171] Additional research has found that coffee seems to boost heart health by reducing calcium buildup in the arteries (an early sign of hardening of the arteries—and a risk for heart disease).[172]

• **It keeps your vision sharp.** Food scientists say you may reap another health benefit from a daily cup of joe: prevention of deteriorating eyesight and possible blindness from retinal degeneration due to glaucoma, aging, and diabetes.[173]

• **It helps prevent diabetes.** Sipping four or more cups of coffee throughout the day (again, a lot—so don't up your intake just because of this study) may reduce your risk of developing type 2 diabetes by 50 percent, says a recent study.[174]

• **It lowers depression.** Researchers found that women who drink two to three cups a day lowered their risk of depression by 15 percent.[175]

• **It reduces your risk of multiple sclerosis (MS).** Johns Hopkins University researchers found that coffee seems to protect against MS.[176] Those people who drank coffee had a lower risk of the autoimmune disease than people who didn't drink it.

• **It helps prevent Alzheimer's disease.** A study published in the *Journal of Alzheimer's Disease* found that drinking at least three cups of coffee a day could prevent the onset of this disease.[177] Plus, a Finnish study found that those who drink three to five cups of coffee a day at midlife have a 65 percent lower risk of developing dementia or Alzheimer's disease in late life than those who drink no coffee at all.[178]

• **It protects against erectile dysfunction.** Caffeinated coffee seems to reduce the risk of erectile dysfunction in men, according to a study from UTHealth School of Public Health, in Houston.[179] Researchers found that men who drink two to three cups of coffee per day were up to 42 percent less likely to report this problem.

• **It boosts athletic performance.** A study from the University of Georgia found that coffee's caffeine could improve endurance in athletes by an average of 24 percent.[180] Roasting and brewing can affect coffee's caffeine levels, found researchers, which could increase or lower athletic performance accordingly.

Healthy Ways to Spice Up Your Coffee

I love my daily cup of coffee. But then I realized there are some easy ways to jazz up your coffee while boosting the content of health-promoting antioxidants. Look beyond the standard add-ins of milk and sugar to jump-start your cup of joe with these healthy alternatives. Add straight to grounds before brewing.

Cardamom: Grind a few cardamom seeds into grounds, and you'll be adding antioxidant minerals like manganese, magnesium, and zinc.

Cayenne: Love spicy foods? Then you'll want to add a dash of this to coffee grounds to give your morning joe a kick. When you do, you'll be enhancing it with antioxidant flavonoids, as well as a small dose of vitamin C, vitamin B_6, potassium, and manganese.

Cinnamon: Add a dash or two to your coffee grounds, and you'll be mixing in the mineral manganese.

Cocoa powder: Mix unsweetened cocoa powder into coffee grounds to add antioxidant flavonoids, as well as fiber, iron, and magnesium. But be sure not to use cocoa powder that's marked "Dutch processed," because this processing can reduce the antioxidant content.[181]

Step Nineteen

Drink tea. Coffee isn't the only hot drink with benefits. There are different types of tea—all with varying health advantages.

Green tea: This tea is made from unwilted leaves that aren't oxidized and contains high concentrations of flavonoids. (It contains little caffeine.)

Numerous studies point to the anti-inflammatory benefits of green tea made from unfermented tea leaves. The reason? Green tea contains an extremely high concentration of powerful antioxidants called catechins, with one of the most potent ones being epigallocatechin gallate, or EGCG. One study found that EGCG might actually block the overproduction of proinflammatory substances in the body, which can trigger cancer.[182] Other studies have linked tea drinking (at least two cups per day) to less heart disease and stroke, lower cholesterol levels, reduced risk of fractures,[183] and even lower rates of cancer.[184]

Black tea: It is produced when tea leaves are wilted, bruised, rolled, and fully oxidized. (Shortly after harvesting, tea leaves begin to wilt and oxidize. During oxidation, chemicals in the leaves are broken down by enzymes, resulting in darkening of the leaves.) It has fewer antioxidants than green tea (the more processed a tea is, the less flavonoids it contains), but it contains more caffeine.

Oolong tea: This is made from wilted, bruised, and partially oxidized leaves, creating an intermediate kind of tea that's midway between green and black teas. It contains a moderate amount of antioxidants and caffeine. It's said to have the body of black tea with the freshness of green tea.

White tea: This tea is made from young leaves or growth buds that have undergone minimal oxidation, meaning it's the least processed of all teas. Because of this, white tea is able to retain its extremely high concentration of antioxidants. It also contains the least caffeine of all teas. It has the most delicate flavor and aroma.

Step Twenty

Eat nuts and seeds. Nuts and seeds (think pumpkin seeds, sunflower seeds, chia seeds, and flaxseeds) are probably some of the healthiest snacks around—why they're integral to a Mediterranean diet. They should also be organic. Munching on nuts and seeds—or nut/seed butter—really does the body and the skin good. One reason: nuts and seeds like almonds and walnuts are high in healthy monounsaturated fats, the same type of health-promoting fats found in olive oil. They're also high in protein and nutrients like fiber, protein, magnesium, potassium, and vitamin E.

Vitamin E is a fat-soluble vitamin that helps prevent oxidative stress to the body. While there are plenty of studies that have shown the benefits of vitamin E, there are two, in particular, that I wanted to highlight. One study, from King's College in London, found that having enough of this key nutrient in your blood protects your lungs from pollution.[185] This makes perfect sense, given that vitamin E is a potent antioxidant that scavenges free radicals, which are created by pollution in the air around us (as well as from a number of other things like the sun's ultraviolet rays, pesticides, and cigarette smoke), to prevent harmful oxidation in the body—and in this case, the lungs.

Research also shows that extra intake of this vitamin (up to 200 IU per day, although the RDA is only 20 IU per day) might actually help regulate the immune system, too, particularly in older adults—helping prevent diseases like pneumonia.[186]

I can attest to the benefits of vitamin E firsthand. When I was in medical school, I ate plenty of nuts, seeds, greens, and healthy fats like avocado (as well as lean meats, beans, and other healthy foods). I knew—from my nutrition classes in graduate school—that vitamin E was just one of the key antioxidants that we need. And, despite the long hours and sometimes overwhelming workload, I rarely got sick. Sometimes, when I was really overloaded, I did take a vitamin E supplement (along with other antioxidants like vitamin C, coenzyme Q10, and glucosamine)—but I really believe that getting your nutrients from food first is always best. You have to be careful of supplementing with vitamin E, in particular, as too much of it can lead to side effects like easy bruising.

One superhealthy nut: Almonds and almond skins have been shown to be a good source of polyphenols (potent antioxidants).[187] In some studies, they've also been found to be a good source of prebiotics, promoting the growth of beneficial microorganisms or bacteria in the intestine,[188] which we've already talked about being so important to overall health of the body and the skin.

These nuts are also a potential beauty food: researchers found that almond-skin extracts—when used in topical formulations—effectively scavenged free radicals while also enhancing skin moisture levels.[189] But I believe eating almonds regularly can achieve similar beauty benefits, because they're such a great source of antioxidants, nutrients, and monounsaturated fats—all of which can result in healthy, glowing skin.

The Secret to Women's Longer Lifespan?

It's well-known that women outlive men (on average by five to six years), but the question is why? Some scientists have found that the female hormone estrogen plays a part.[190]

According to the research, estrogen increases blood stem cells in female mice and helps them regenerate brain stem cells faster than male mice. And male mice lived longer, too, when given estrogen supplements.

Another study, from Boston University School of Medicine, found that the ability to have children later in life (after the age of thirty-three) is linked to longevity in women.[191] Researchers believe this ability suggests a reproductive system—which is fueled by estrogen and other hormones—that simply ages at a slower pace. Women, they say, who give birth after thirty-three are twice as likely to live to ninety-five or older, compared with those who had their last child by the age of twenty-nine.

Other experts believe, however, that it's not just estrogen that plays a role; it may be that women are more prone to iron deficiency because of their periods—and iron, while a key mineral, produces free radicals that contribute to aging and disease.[192] So less iron may mean less overall free-radical damage. Women are also more likely to take better care of themselves and have healthy social networks—both of which contribute to a longer lifespan.

What to Eat for Silky, Shiny Hair

We've discussed so much about health of the body and the skin. But we haven't talked about another important healthy beauty topic: hair.

We're bombarded with ads for the latest hair products—from shampoos to gravity-defying gels—designed to give you gorgeous, enviable locks. But the part of the great-hair-day story that is often left out is how what you eat affects how your hair looks.

Abbie*, one of my patients, was trying to lose weight on a rice-cake-and-water diet for months. She came in to see me because she was losing her hair. I talked with her about the importance of eating a diverse, healthy Mediterranean-style diet. Within just weeks of eating healthier, her hair stopped falling out, and within months, she saw her hair growing back.

Even though hair is technically "dead" (it's made up of dead cells composed of keratin, a fibrous protein, and has no blood, nerves, or muscles), it's actually the second-fastest-growing type of cell in your body (bone marrow is the first).

It all starts from the follicle: at the base of the follicle is the papilla, from which hair grows. Capillaries surrounding the follicles (each follicle has its own blood supply) nourish the cell production and growth of each individual strand. Why this is important: if you aren't eating a healthy diet—with enough key nutrients and protein—your hair follicle won't be nourished, and your hair will look lackluster and might even fall out.

Hormonal fluctuations and stress—both emotional and physical—can also affect the density and shine of your locks.

So then, what should you be eating for shiny, lustrous locks? Start with these Mediterranean staples:

Nuts: You may have heard about the benefits of biotin for hair health in a shampoo ad, or read in a magazine that taking biotin supplements can make your hair grow faster (and your nails stronger). There is some truth to this. Biotin is a B vitamin essential for hair growth and overall scalp health. Our bodies make their own biotin in the intestines, and it's also found in many common foods. A biotin deficiency is therefore very rare, so supplements are usually unnecessary if you're eating a balanced diet that includes some high-biotin foods.

Peanuts are a great choice, as they're also high in B vitamins and folate, which contribute to healthy hair. Other biotin-rich foods are almonds, sweet potatoes, eggs, onions, and oats. Salmon has a small amount of biotin, but it's still a good option, as it's key to the Mediterranean diet.

Oranges and strawberries: Juicy citrus fruits often get the credit as the best vitamin C–packed fruit, but just eight strawberries deliver 100 percent of your daily needs (something most people don't realize). Strawberries are a juicy, delicious source of vitamin C, which is largely responsible for the health of collagen.

Hair follicles require collagen, a structural fiber, for optimal growth. Even minor vitamin C deficiencies can lead to dry, splitting hair that breaks easily, so eating vitamin C–rich foods like strawberries, oranges, grapefruit, kiwifruit, red and green bell peppers, kale, broccoli, papaya, and pineapple can all help you grow stronger, more resilient strands.

Beans and legumes: Legumes, particularly lentils, are especially high in both folate and iron, two powerful nutrients that nourish your mane. Folate is a B vitamin that aids the creation of red blood cells; iron helps those blood cells carry oxygen and nutrients to all body cells. With iron deficiency, a condition known as anemia, cells can't get enough oxygen to function properly. The result can be devastating to the whole body, causing weakness, fatigue, and in some cases, even hair loss. So load up on iron-rich lentils for sturdy tresses—and if you're a premenopausal woman, consider taking a multivitamin that contains iron to replace iron lost during menstruation. Other good non-red-meat sources of iron include fish (sardines, halibut, haddock, salmon, and tuna); beans (lima beans, red kidney beans, split peas); and pumpkin, sesame, or squash seeds.

In addition to providing zinc and folate (nutrients that promote hair health), chickpeas are a great vegetarian source of iron-rich protein, an important combination for hair growth and repair. Because hair gets its structure from hardened proteins called keratin, people who don't have enough protein in their diet experience slower growth and weaker strands. To increase the absorption of iron from chickpeas, couple with a vitamin C–rich food such as tomatoes, bell peppers, or citrus fruit.

Chicken: Protein is critical to healthy hair—and skinless chicken breast is another healthy source of protein. It's rich in B vitamins (like folate, B6, and B12) that maintain healthy hair. These vitamins play an important role in the creation of red blood cells, which carry oxygen and nutrients to all body cells, including those of the scalp, follicles, and growing hair. When the body is deprived of B vitamins, the cells can starve, causing shedding, slow growth, or weak strands that are prone to breaking.

Propolis: While not your typical "food," propolis—a resin-like material that honeybees use to patch holes in their hives—has been found to encourage hair growth. Researchers believe its benefits are a result of its anti-inflammatory and antioxidant properties.[193]

➔ **Where do you go from here?** Put these healthy diet strategies into practice, and I guarantee that you'll be on your way to a healthy body and healthy skin for years to come. Diet is the foundation for everything that relates to your body. Don't get discouraged, though, if you can't do all of them at once. The best way to institute healthy eating is to incorporate one or two (or even three) strategies into your life for twenty-one days, the amount of time it takes for a habit to become ingrained. Then you can incorporate more strategies as you're ready to take another step on your journey toward health and longevity—and inner and outer beauty.

Remember: health is not a race. Slow and steady good habits, particularly when it comes to your diet, are what wins in the end. Before you move on to the next chapter, look back at your list of things that you want to change about your body and your skin, and see how this chapter can help you make those things happen.

In the words of Virginia Woolf, remember that "One cannot think well, love well, sleep well, if one has not dined well."

CHAPTER 2

Cultivate Inner Peace and Spirituality

"If you want to conquer the anxiety of life, live in the moment, live in the breath."

~ Zig Ziglar

My patient Michael* is a trial attorney and was under a lot of stress. He noticed that every time he had a big trial case, his psoriasis would get considerably worse, with red and white, patchy, scaling skin all over his body. It was really bothering him, but as he worked long hours, he didn't think that he had the time to address it. Michael's wife finally couldn't stand listening to him complain about it anymore and told him to see a dermatologist. That's when Michael booked an appointment with me.

When Michael came into my office, he was stressed and anxious, and his psoriasis was in full flare-up mode. I spoke to him about his condition and how we could treat it with prescription medication. But I also spoke to him about the importance of healthy eating, stress-reduction techniques, exercise, and taking better care of himself in general. Since psoriasis is a chronic, immune-mediated disease, there has been a great deal of research[194] showing the benefits of a healthy lifestyle[195]—including stress management and an anti-inflammatory Mediterranean-style diet[196]—in reducing the symptoms and flare-ups.

When Michael came back for his follow-up several months later, he looked like a whole different person. He explained that he had thought a lot about what I said and that it made a big impression on him. He thanked me for taking the time to address more than just his psoriasis.

Michael discovered that there was a gym in his work building—and started exercising thirty minutes several days a week. He also started meditating during his lunch hour instead of watching television shows on his computer. He explained that not only did his skin improve but also his clarity of thinking. He felt like he was more productive at work.

Like Michael, we all experience stress: no one is immune. It's a normal, almost expected, part of life today thanks to busy family lives, work, being connected to our smartphones and computers 24/7, financial ups and downs, relationship issues, health issues, and negative thinking. Pretty much everything in our too-busy lives can trigger stress—both emotional and physical. Even good experiences like running a race, giving a speech, or celebrating a big event can cause stress.

What's common in all these situations is that they require a response from us (also called the body's stress response). This is the body's natural alarm system—the so-called "flight or fight" response—that prepares us to fight a perceived stressor or run from it.

This stress response can be short-lived, which—if minor—doesn't take a great physical toll on us because our bodies have a chance to recover. But sudden major "acute" stressors—emotional (like explosive anger) or physical (like an earthquake)—can trigger heart attacks and even sudden death.[197]

Stress responses can also be episodic, where the response remains for a longer period of time and to a greater degree; this is what triggers a greater health toll on the body. The body's stress response can also be chronic (the worst), in which there is very little recuperation time and a lot of wear and tear on our body and mind over time.

When we experience long-term chronic stress (which so many of us are experiencing now in modern life), the health of our body and of our skin suffers. Understanding how stress affects the body and the skin will help you understand how and why stress triggers problems like acne and skin rashes, causes illness and chronic disease, and affects our longevity.

My patients always ask me why (and how) I always seem to be so upbeat, happy, and grounded all the time. If only they knew! I get frazzled just as much as the next person, but I've learned to get a handle on it by meditating every morning for about ten to fifteen minutes and before bed at night for the same amount of time. (Several times a week, though, I set aside thirty minutes to meditate before bed. I sit on the edge of my bed to do this instead of lying down to avoid falling asleep.) I also try to shut my office door for ten minutes during my lunchtime so I can sit at my desk and meditate. I find that it keeps me grounded throughout the day.

I also try to do yoga several times a week. I find it beneficial both physically and mentally. The key, though, is to find what works for you—and incorporate it into your life. That's what this chapter is all about.

How Stress Affects the Body and the Skin

Consider these effects of stress on health:[198]

• **43 percent** of all adults suffer adverse health effects from stress.

• **75–90 percent** of all doctor's office visits are for stress-related ailments and complaints.

• **$300 billion or more** is what stress costs American industry annually (the Occupational Safety and Health Administration, or OSHA, has declared stress a hazard of the workplace).

• **40 percent** of adults lie awake at night because of stress.[199]

When the body encounters a perceived stressor—be it a looming deadline, a fight with a spouse, or the death of a loved one—it gets ready for action. The hypothalamus (the part of the brain responsible for hormone production) communicates with the adrenal glands (situated above the kidneys), alerting them to pump out stress hormones like corticotropin-releasing hormone (CRH), glucocorticoids like cortisol, and epinephrine (adrenaline). These hormones (the most well-known of which is cortisol) help get the body ready to react.

When these hormones are released, the liver produces more glucose, or blood sugar, to provide the body with extra energy to help you react to the problem and to prepare the body to deal with it. Our muscles tense up as the body's way of guarding against injury and pain. We also start to breathe rapidly. We're entering full-on panic mode.

These stress hormones also cause an increase in heart rate and stronger contractions of the heart muscle. The blood vessels that direct blood to the large muscles and the heart dilate, increasing the amount of blood being pumped though the body. The result is increased blood pressure.

Under stress, your body also releases a protein called neuropeptide S or NPS, which decreases sleep and increases alertness. The body is essentially keeping you awake and alert to face the danger it senses. So if you wonder why you're tossing and turning—or waking up in the middle of the night and having trouble going back to sleep—stress is the culprit. (Taking a sleeping pill without addressing the underlying causes of stress will wear down the body, triggering long-term health problems down the road.)

The skin, it turns out, also becomes stressed.[200] Neurotransmitters (brain chemicals that communicate information throughout our brain and body) are released, triggering stress-related responses and inflammation in the skin. The result: skin problems like acne, eczema, psoriasis, and dermatitis. The inflammation—along with free-radical formation—that stress causes can also contribute to premature aging of the skin, including wrinkles; dry, rough skin; and hyperpigmentation.

Under stress, the skin's barrier function is also compromised, allowing irritants to enter and moisture to escape (why stressed skin gets dry, rough, and dull).

All these reactions in the body can trigger both emotional and physical problems[201]—particularly when they're being activated for long periods of time. Long-term stress has been linked to depression;[202] anxiety; headaches;[203] heart attacks;[204] stroke; hypertension; type 2 diabetes;[205] a depressed immune system; cancer; autoimmune diseases like rheumatoid arthritis[206] and multiple sclerosis; degenerative neurological disorders like Parkinson's disease;[207] a loss of concentration and memory; fatigue and insomnia; and gastrointestinal disturbances like constipation, ulcers, irritable bowel syndrome (IBS), and colitis.[208]

Long term, scientists believe that too much chronic stress can reduce our lifespan by causing age-related deterioration in our bodies. In a nutshell: stress causes us to age faster. In one experiment with fruit flies, scientists found that the fruit flies that were resistant to stress—with all its effects on the body—actually lived longer than those who weren't resistant to stress.[209]

Some scientists are also studying the relationship between psychological stress and aging.[210] One group of scientists found is that people under extreme psychological stress have shortened telomeres, when compared to those not under extreme psychological stress. These telomeres exist in each of our cells and hold the secrets to our DNA and genetic data, including how we age. Telomeres have been compared with the plastic tips on shoelaces,[211] because they keep the ends of chromosomes (the twisted, double-stranded molecules of DNA that exist in the nucleus of each cell in our body) from fraying and sticking to each other, which could destroy or scramble an organism's genetic information.

The younger you are, the longer these telomeres are. But each time a cell divides as we get older, these telomeres get shorter. Oxidative stress and inflammation can also speed up the shortening of these telomeres. Lifestyle factors such as obesity, cigarette smoking, and consumption of sugary food and drinks have all been linked to people having shorter telomeres.[212]

When telomeres get too short, the cell can no longer divide; it becomes inactive, or it dies. Tissue can't regenerate anymore. This shortening process or "internal clock"[213] is associated with aging, some cancers (specifically bladder, bone, head and neck, kidney, lung, and pancreatic[214]), and a higher risk of death.[215]

Preliminary research has also shown that cancer cells somehow seem to reprogram these telomeres, enabling the cancer cells to proliferate and become virtually immortal.[216] It's a fascinating area of health research today—and I believe we've just started to see how important these telomeres are to every single aspect of our health.

What we know for sure now is that reducing stress and living a healthy life can help keep telomeres longer—as can following a Mediterranean diet. One study, published in *BMJ*, found that eating plenty of vegetables, fruits, legumes, unrefined grains, fish, and olive oil, characteristic of a Mediterranean diet, was "significantly associated with longer telomeres."[217] Regular practice of transcendental meditation has also been shown to stimulate genes to produce telomerase,[218] which adds molecules to the ends of telomeres to protect them from deteriorating.

Stress and the skin: There's no question that stress affects the skin, and for good reason: the skin is the primary sensing organ for external stressors, including heat, cold, pain, and tension.[219] Plenty of research has been done to back this up. Some researchers have found that the brain, in turn, responds to these signals, which can influence the stress response in the skin.[220] Increased perspiration, constriction of blood vessels, and decreased blood flow to the skin all occur when the body is under stress.[221]

Stress has been shown to have direct effects on the skin in the form of rashes, hives, acne, psoriasis, and atopic dermatitis. Researchers believe this may be a result of impaired skin barrier function (the skin's barrier helps hold in moisture, keeping skin hydrated).[222] Stress has also been associated with slower wound healing[223] and increased susceptibility to infections.[224] It may also prompt your hair to fall out; stress has been linked to the autoimmune condition alopecia areata, which causes hair loss.[225]

Researchers have also found that long-term stress can increase DNA damage to the skin and interfere with DNA repair, both of which can trigger premature aging of the skin. Stress has also been shown to accelerate the growth and progression of skin cancer.[226] And what's more: research shows that chronic psychological stress results in a shortening of the telomeres that we've talked about at a much more rapid pace[227]—which triggers aging of the skin.

Sleeplessness and loss of sleep is also a form of stress on the body and can impact the skin. One study found that poor sleepers have increased fine lines, uneven pigmentation, and reduced elasticity in their skin.[228]

Stress and vitamin C: Stress—especially if it's intense and prolonged—rapidly depletes vitamin C, an antioxidant, from the body. (One of the highest concentrations of vitamin C in the body is in the adrenal glands, which play a central role in dealing with stress.) Smoking also depletes vitamin C from the body.

So it's not surprising that vitamin C helps reduce both the psychological and physical effects of stress. This vitamin seems to counteract or even prevent secretion of the key stress hormone, cortisol, that's responsible for triggering the "flight or fight" response to stress.[229] As an antioxidant, vitamin C is also responsible for protecting blood vessels, helping create the skin-firming protein collagen, and supporting the immune system. (This explains why smokers have advanced premature skin aging, as well as an increased propensity for vascular disease.[230])

Whatever you do, be sure to get enough vitamin C on a daily basis. You can find this key nutrient in fresh, uncooked fruits like oranges, papayas, and strawberries and in vegetables like red and green peppers, broccoli, brussels sprouts, and asparagus.

How We React to Stress

When we're under stress and functioning in full-on crisis mode, we slack off on healthy habits such as getting enough sleep, exercising, and eating a healthy diet. A diet that contains empty calories and is lacking in vitamins, minerals, and antioxidants can cause you to have low mental and physical energy.

This self-neglect can further fuel stress. With diet, for example, when we're under stress, our bodies have elevated levels of the stress hormone cortisol—something that triggers our sugar and carbohydrate cravings. (Ever wonder why you reach for cookies, candy, and sweets when you're stressed? It has nothing to do with willpower; it has everything to do with stress.)

If the stress is short-lived, the effects aren't severe. But when the stress is chronic, this sugar can make us more reactive to stress and more predisposed to diseases like diabetes and obesity, as well as to premature aging. Processed foods in general (which include so many of the foods we reach for during stress) can put strain on the body—and even trigger addictive eating.[231] These foods, as well as the stress that causes us to crave them, trigger the production of damaging and aging free radicals.

Many of us also tend to react to stress with feelings of being overwhelmed and helpless. It's important to be able to recognize the causes of stress in our lives and to manage them. Some stressors cannot be eliminated, though, and this is when our frame of mind is important: we *can* control how we react to a situation that's beyond our control. Don't let a difficult person or situation steal your peace.

How we perceive a situation, as well as how we react, makes a difference in whether we're relaxed or we trigger our stress response. We've all seen an example of this when stuck in a traffic jam. Some people react with anger and aggression over being made late for work or an appointment, and others are able to sit back and enjoy the music and accept the possibility of being late. With practice, we can shape our natural tendencies and react to things differently.

Eat to Beat Stress

A well-balanced diet can help you function your best during times of stress. Some steps to avoid unhealthy stress-induced eating habits include:

✓ **Prepare your pantry.** If you tend to reach for the fastest meal while under stress, then stock your kitchen with quick, healthy food options. This can include fruits, vegetables, and healthy dips. You can also cook extra portions of healthy meals that can be quickly reheated. Don't buy foods you know are unhealthy, so they won't be an option during stressful times.

✓ **Keep healthy restaurants on speed dial.** Knowing ahead of time where the healthy restaurant options are in your area can help you avoid unhealthy eating habits. Also, take a look at the menus at these restaurants so you have healthy standbys when you're in a rush.

✓ **Practice portion control.** If you have cravings or cannot cut out all unhealthy food, you may want to cut back the amount you consume and practice portion control. Remember to practice moderation.

✓ **Swap out unhealthy snacks.** I'm all too familiar with the sugar and processed-food cravings that accompany stress, but stopping these anxiety-provoked binges before they start will keep your energy and mood up—and keep your skin radiant and more youthful looking. Instead, try an apple with a nut or seed butter, homemade trail mix, or string cheese and crackers.

The key with stress-busting snacks is keeping the junk out of your home and your office—and having the healthy options on hand for those stress-induced munchies.

Take a Deep Breath...and Stop Smoking

Taking long, deep breaths in and out...in and out...is a common relaxation practice. It's also common practice for smokers—and taking a break from the craziness of life to do this outdoors is how smokers begin to associate smoking with relaxation. This is why so many smokers reach for a cigarette when they're stressed—and why once this habit gets engrained (and the nicotine addiction sets in), it's so hard to break.

The chemicals in smoke: While the relaxation effect is good in theory, all those chemicals you're breathing into your body (more than seven thousand altogether![232]) are simply no good. Hundreds of these chemicals have been proven toxic, and about seventy are known to cause cancer, like formaldehyde, benzene (found in gasoline), polonium 210 (radioactive), and vinyl chloride (used to make pipes).[233] Plus, every one of these chemicals can create the formation of free radicals in the body—which contributes to premature aging of the body and the skin.[234]

Secondhand smoke is also toxic. This smokes contains the same seven thousand chemicals that smokers expose themselves to when smoking. Secondhand cigarette smoke can cause frequent and severe asthma attacks, respiratory infections, ear infections, sudden infant death syndrome, heart disease, stroke, and lung cancer.[235] One particularly concerning study found that nonsmokers who sat in a car with a smoker for just one hour (even with the windows slightly open) had significantly increased levels of carcinogens and other toxins—associated with cancer, heart disease, and lung disease—in their urine.[236]

Even third-hand smoke—the smoke pollutants that remain in an indoor environment on surfaces or in dust where smokers have smoked (as in a home or in a car)—is dangerous. One group of researchers found that these indoor surfaces represent "a hidden reservoir" of third-hand smoke pollutants that could be "reemitted long after the cessation of active smoking."[237] This is extremely concerning.

Bottom line: commit to quit. Relaxation techniques like yoga, meditation, and walking outdoors may help you cope with the stresses of daily life—so you don't want to reach for that cigarette when the going gets tough (or tougher).

The Happiness Factor

So many of us underestimate the value of happiness in our lives. But the truth is that by following our hearts and taking time to truly enjoy every moment of every day, we can make a huge impact on our happiness and on our health. One of my favorite sayings is this one:

> *"I have chosen to be happy because it is good for my health." (Voltaire)*

How true this is! Just feeling positive—and looking at life from a glass-half-full perspective—can do wonders for your happiness. A big part of this is making the choice to be happy and to not let the bad things in life get you down. Viktor Frankl, in *Man's Search for Meaning*, touches on how a positive attitude allows a person to endure suffering and disappointments and can enhance satisfaction. A negative attitude, however, can worsen pain or disappointment and undermine satisfaction.

We all have the freedom to choose how we'll respond to a situation—and how we approach each situation in our lives (with either a positive or a negative attitude) helps shape the meaning of our lives.

Research shows that staying positive and happy can boost one's health. One study found that people who are cheerful and positive in the face of stress have lower levels of inflammation in the body.[238] Failing to maintain a positive, happy outlook had the opposite effect: elevated levels of disease-triggering inflammation, particularly in women.

Importance of friends, family, and loved ones: One way to take positive steps toward happiness is through friends and family: numerous studies have shown that healthy relationships are good for us emotionally and physically. People with happy relationships—and an overall positive view of life—are less stressed overall and have a better immune system,[239] decreased health issues (like heart disease), lower levels of stress, and increased longevity.[240]

In fact, one study found that just the act of hugging someone can boost your health. Researchers from Carnegie Mellon University found that greater social support and frequent hugs protect stressed people from illness and disease—and when social people do get sick, their strong social network protects them from more severe illness symptoms.[241]

If you're married or in a close personal relationship, sex can help reduce stress, too—and even make you look five to seven years younger.[242] This is the result of the secretion, during sex, of the human growth hormone or HGH (a hormone that plays a key role in boosting skin elasticity); oxytocin (the hormone that lowers the stress hormone, cortisol); and endorphins (natural anxiety busters and painkillers that make you feel good and help you get a good night's sleep).

I would also say that people who are happier are more beautiful: they have a natural glow about them—as well as an indescribable energy—that radiates from the inside out to the skin.

Compelling research shows that these positive, happy emotions and an overall enjoyment of life contribute to better health and a longer lifespan.[243] One Dutch study found that just cheerfulness helped older people live almost 7.5 years longer.[244]

In compelling research conducted by University of Illinois, this link among happiness, health, and longevity is stronger than the data linking obesity to reduced longevity.[245] One possible reason for this link between happiness and health: researchers have found that being happy increases our antibodies—critical proteins utilized by the immune system to fight off viruses, bacteria, and more—by a whopping 50 percent.[246]

Daily news intake and anxiety: There are so many stress-provoking stories in the news today that it's no wonder people are so full of stress and depression. While it's important to stay informed, too much news viewing has been shown to cause stress and anxiety. Try avoiding media for a few days each month—and always at least an hour before going to bed each night—and see how you feel.

When it comes to what's going on in the world—or even in just our own lives—I've found that these words (repeated often or pasted up on a note by your desk or on your fridge) can often help:

"God, grant me the serenity to accept the things I cannot change, the courage to change the things I can, and the wisdom to know the difference." (Reinhold Niebuhr)

Benefits of mindfulness meditation: Mindfulness meditation—a form of meditation designed to develop the skill of paying attention to our inner and outer experiences with acceptance, patience, and compassion[247]—can also help get rid of the negative, anxiety-provoking thoughts, clearing the way for happiness. Mindfulness meditation has been shown in studies to improve anxiety, depression, and pain (often a side effect of chronic stress).[248] I advise all my patients to try to take up meditation if they can. Not only does it help relieve stress and anxiety, but it can also help you tune into your body and what it's telling you through symptoms, fatigue, cravings, and yearnings. As the well-known Hindu scripture, the Bhagavad Gita, says: "With a quiet mind, seek harmony within yourself."

Link between regular exercise and less stress: Another habit that can help make you feel happier: regular exercise. Working out regularly has been shown to mimic the effects of antidepressants on the brain. The reason: when you exercise, the body releases endorphins, chemicals secreted by the hypothalamus. When these endorphins are released, they lock onto special receptor cells (called opioid receptors, because opiates also fit them), where they block the transmission of pain signals and also produce a euphoric feeling (just like opiates do).[249] Exercise has also been shown to improve sleep—enough of which can make anyone's outlook on the world rosier.

Having a hard time staying happy when everything seems to be falling apart around you? Try visualization, where you imagine a scene that is pleasing to you. When we vividly picture a pleasing activity, our brain believes it's experiencing what we're visualizing, shifting our attention and helping clear negative thoughts.

How to Practice Mindfulness Meditation

Consistent daily practice of mindfulness meditation has been shown to calm the mind and allow us to better face the stressors in our lives. It's based on noticing the moment when our awareness connects with our present situation (we want to deliberately cultivate this kind of simple awareness!).

As the classic Chinese text, the Tao Te Ching, says: "Close the door and shut out the senses. Do this and you will never be exhausted." The benefit of meditation is that we become more synchronized in body and mind and being to relate to our world in a less distracted and more wakeful way. This more balanced approach to life manifests itself in how we act every day—and how we look, too. So many of my stressed patients come in with stressed skin and look years older than their actual age. Those of my patients who meditate regularly exude a calmer, more radiant glow from their skin. They look younger, too.

To practice mindfulness meditation, sit in a comfortable spot and keep your eyes open in a soft downward gaze, looking four to six feet on the floor in front of you. (The idea is that you're not shutting down your awareness of the space around you, but you are relaxing your focus somewhat.) Ideally, you want to sit with your back straight—and in a lotus or half-lotus posture (though this isn't necessary), where you're sitting cross-legged with the feet placed on opposing thighs. The tips of the thumb and index finger are touching, forming a circle, with the back of the hand resting on the lower thighs and the palm open and inward to the heart (this is the "knowledge" position).

Now, it's time to focus on your breathing—in and out. (You want your awareness to become connected to your breath.) Follow the physical sensations of the breath as it moves in and out of the body. Continually bring your mind's attention to the present, and your breath, without drifting into concerns about the past or future. If your mind does drift to thoughts about your day and your life (this is normal!), simply bring it back to the present, peacefully and without judgment.

It's important not to repress thoughts or follow them. Just let them be as they are, notice them, and then return your attention to your breath. The Buddhist meditation master Chögyam Trungpa Rinpoche used to say that when you are sitting like this, you have a flat bottom, and your thoughts also have a flat bottom. Before, your thoughts had little wings and were flying all around and taking you with them—but now your body is settled, and your mental activity will settle down as well.

Some people find it helpful to have a mantra (a single word or sound like "ohm") or an image to focus on. Then every time your mind drifts, you simply refocus it with your mantra or visual image. Or you can just make the breath your image and your mantra.

According to some research, stress often causes unproductive worries and distracting thoughts that mindfulness meditation (learning to be calm in the moment and to quell unproductive thoughts) can help control.[250]

Keep in mind that, as with learning any new skill, practice is key. The art of pushing aside all the thoughts in your brain to focus on your breath *will* become a little easier each time you do it.

How to Breathe to Relieve Stress

"But I know how to breathe," is probably most people's response when they hear they need to learn how to really breathe—how a baby or young child breathes. This is called diaphragmatic breathing.

The diaphragm—called the most efficient muscle of breathing—is the large dome-shaped muscle located at the base of the lungs. Deep diaphragmatic breathing (slow breathing from this muscle)—as opposed to shallow breathing from the chest (how most of us breathe, a hallmark of anxiety)—has been used for thousands of years as a way to enhance health and even spiritual practices.

This is how we breathe from the time we're born—but then our breaths become more shallow as we get older and start to experience stress (and in the process, forget how to breathe).

Also called yoga breathing, diaphragmatic breathing is both a form of meditation and a preparation for deep meditation—and has been shown to reduce stress and treat depression, anxiety, and even post-traumatic stress disorder (PTSD).[251]

Diaphragmatic breathing can also strengthen the diaphragm (it *is* a muscle, so it needs to be worked to be strengthened), slow your breathing rate (and lessen your anxiety), decrease oxygen demand on the body, increase lymphatic flow to strengthen the immune system, and use less effort and energy to breathe.[252]

To perform diaphragmatic breathing:[253]

1. Find a quiet place, get comfortable, and start by relaxing your head, neck, and shoulders. You can lie on your back on a flat surface or in bed, with your knees bent and your head supported. You can use a pillow under your knees to support your legs. (You can also do this sitting in a chair with your knees bent and your feet on the floor, head and neck relaxed.)

2. Place one hand on your upper chest and the other just below your rib cage. This will allow you to feel your diaphragm move as you breathe.

3. Breathe in slowly through your nose so that your stomach moves out against your hand. This hand on your chest should remain as still as possible.

4. Tighten your stomach muscles, letting them fall inward as you exhale through pursed lips. Again, the hand on your upper chest should remain as still as possible.

You should try to practice this breathing for five to ten minutes, three to four times per day.

The Eight Habits of Happy People

I've read so much about what makes happy people happy and the things they do on a daily basis that makes them so joyful. What I know is this: being cheerful is contagious—for you (you want to be happy more and more) and for everyone else around you (it's hard not to smile when someone else smiles at you!).

It also brings a natural radiance and beauty to your face that can't be mimicked by any skin creams or treatments. Happy people are beautiful people. This is what I call truly natural beauty.

Here, then, are the habits of happy people. Try them; they're contagious!

✓ **Smile.** Smiling makes you happy on the inside. It lights up your face and makes others happy to be around you. There's a natural beauty in those who smile a lot.

✓ **Appreciate the simple things in the everyday.** Big victories and events shouldn't be the focus in life. It's the small victories and pleasures that we also should be finding joy in. Many times these small things are around us every day; they're not something to be gotten or achieved or bought. If we stop chasing happiness, we will realize that opportunities for fun and meaningfulness are all around us. This is why I love this quote from Frederick Keonig:

"We tend to forget that happiness doesn't come as a result of getting something we don't have, but rather of recognizing and appreciating what we do have."

✓ **See the glass as half full.** As hard as it is to look at life from the bright side, doing so will make you happier. In fact, being positive has been linked to a healthier heart, too.[254]

✓ **Take time to relax.** The happiest people are those who take regular breaks from daily stress. Whether it be regular meditation, yoga, exercise, daily walks, or even just taking time for yourself to do something you enjoy, taking a break from the grind *will* make you happier.

✓ **Be resilient.** Knowing how to get back on track when life doesn't go according to plan is key to happy people's cheerfulness.

✓ **Do good—for others and for the world.** The sense of helping others and the world at large gives happy people what's been called a "helper's high" and seems to help protect them against depression.

✓ **Cultivate your spiritual side.** Spirituality, as I also say later in this book, gives you a sense that there's something greater in the world than just you. This is a humbling way to think, and it seems to help happy people shrug off the not-so-great things that happen in life. Cultivating spirituality has also been shown to be good for your health: one study found that a sense of spirituality can help reduce depression and nurture hope.[255]

✓ **Spend time with other people.** Happy people are those who have strong social ties and close family and friends. Very simply, the more social you are, the happier you'll be.

Pets help make people happy, too, because they provide meaningful social support.[256] In one study, pet owners were found to have higher self-esteem, feel less lonely, be less fearful, and be more socially outgoing[257]—all factors that can make one less stressed and more happy. These same pet owners had a greater sense of belongingness, meaningful existence, and control over their lives. I can see this firsthand in my own life; my two dogs, Lexington and Madison, are integral parts of our family life. They add so much daily pleasure and love, and they make our family smile and laugh.

But excluding everything else, just making it a habit to count your blessings on a daily basis can help make you happier. Make a list if you have to, every day, of the five to ten things that bring you happiness. You might just find your outlook shifting for the better.

There are four cardinal virtues—outlined by Lao Tzu in the Tao Te Ching—that closely mimic the habits of happy people: reverence for all life, natural sincerity, gentleness, and supportiveness. According to Lao Tzu, it is through these principles that we align spiritually and, in turn, receive universal guidance and support. In this way, we are able to cultivate true inner peace. I would also say, it is through these principles that we can cultivate true happiness.

Stress and Weight Gain: The Truth

Turns out there's a lot of truth behind the whole idea of stress eating—and it may not have anything to do with our willpower (or lack of it).

In the short term, stress can shut down appetite.[258] When under stress, the hypothalamus produces a corticotropin-releasing hormone, which suppresses hunger. Adrenaline, produced by the adrenal glands, also temporarily puts eating on hold. But if stress persists, then this normal stress response goes a bit haywire.

Some researchers have found that chronic stress can actually increase appetite—thanks to the hormone cortisol.[259] And it's not healthy fruits and veggies that we crave; it's sugar and fat like chocolate-chip cookies and greasy cheeseburgers. A group of scientists at the University of California San Francisco found that this desire for comfort foods may be a biological way of feeding the body enough energy to sustain the fight-or-flight response long term.[260]

Additional research also shows that highly processed foods—like candy, pizza, french fries, and potato chips—in turn, can fuel addictive eating.[261] So what happens is a vicious cycle of binging and addictive eating that can challenge even those with the strongest willpower. This doesn't come as a surprise as so many of us can relate to this!

Eating this way over the long haul can pack on pounds, particularly in the abdominal area.[262] And abdominal obesity can lead to cardiovascular disease, type 2 diabetes, and stroke.

Obesity can affect the skin as well. It increases:

• **Water loss from the skin** (resulting in dry skin that has less ability to repair wounds)

• **Susceptibility to acne** (thanks to higher-than-normal levels of hormones circulating in the body; hormones are stored in fat)

• **Sweating** (due to the thick layers of fat under the skin)

• **Fluid buildup in the skin** (due to slowed lymphatic flow through the body)[263]

Obesity can also aggravate skin conditions like psoriasis and skin infections.

So the goal needs to be, first, finding ways to reduce your stress and, second, finding new ways to eat for stress—and energy. The Mediterranean diet is a good place to start.

Complementary and Alternative Therapies

These therapies—like meditation, visualization, and breath work, which I have already briefly discussed—can be a beneficial addition to a healthy lifestyle that includes a Mediterranean diet and regular exercise. All work to reduce anxiety and keep you feeling calmer. I see this in my patients who regularly follow these healthy-living strategies. Some research also shows that these therapies, also referred to as complementary and alternative therapies, can have antiaging benefits and improve overall health.[264] What's more, these stress-busting techniques can also boost immune functioning.[265]

Healing Touch

Acupressure and acupuncture: Both developed over five thousand years ago as a part of traditional Chinese medicine (also referred to as TCM). They both involve precise finger placement and pressure—or with needles, in acupuncture—on specific body points or meridians. In Asian medical philosophy, manipulation of these points with pressure or needles can improve blood flow, healing, and tension and unblock or increase vital qi (pronounced "chee") energy. It's believed that balancing the meridians allows healing energy to flow more freely in the body.

Acupressure and acupuncture can be used to relieve pain and muscle tension,[266] to promote relaxation, and to alleviate sexual dysfunction[267] and infertility.[268] Studies have shown that they can also help prevent nausea from motion sickness,[269] decrease menstrual cramps,[270] and assist in quitting smoking.[271]

Research also shows that walking on river-stone paths—which activates acupressure points on the soles of the feet—can relieve pain, improve sleep, increase balance, lower blood pressure, and improve overall physical and mental wellness.[272]

– **Acupuncture for healthier skin** For thousands of years, acupuncture has been used to treat disorders of the skin, as well as disorders of the body. For skin disorders, acupuncture points are stimulated along the arms, legs, and torso.[273]

Several small studies have been conducted showing its benefits, but it hasn't been until recently that scientists have conducted a thorough analysis of research on the benefits of acupuncture in the treatment of skin problems like dermatitis, hives, itchy skin, excessive sweating (or hyperhidrosis), pigmentation, and even facial elasticity.[274]

These researchers—from the University of California, Davis—have found that, indeed, acupuncture did improve results in patients when used as the primary treatment.

The Chinese have also used acupuncture and acupressure for centuries as a beauty treatment to enhance facial muscle tone and to boost facial circulation, which helps improve the appearance of the skin and lessens wrinkles.

Massage therapy: We've probably all enjoyed a good massage at one point or another—and experienced firsthand its relaxing results. There are many different types of massage therapy, from Swedish massage (designed to promote relaxation) to sports massage (more of a therapeutic massage designed to knead trouble spots). There's even facial massage to help relieve tension and stress in the skin.

There's evidence showing measurable health benefits from all types of massage, given that they all involve the manipulation of the muscles and soft tissues. Massage has been shown to help reduce pain,[275] speed recovery after injury,[276] increase flexibility,[277] loosen muscles,[278] boost relaxation,[279] and reduce stress.[280] Studies have shown that massage can lower heart rate and blood pressure,[281] increase circulation[282] and lymphatic flow,[283] improve immune function,[284] lower the level of stress hormones like cortisol,[285] and increase the production of endorphins.[286]

Osteopathy: Osteopathy is a form of medicine—founded by Andrew Taylor Still in 1874—that focuses on total-body, or holistic, health. This is the form of medicine that I practice. I believe that the body functions as an integral unit, not as a collection of separate parts.[287] Osteopathic doctors like me place an emphasis on self-healing and preventive medicine.

Osteopathic physicians are also trained in osteopathic manipulative treatment or hands-on care to diagnose, treat, and prevent illness or injury. The techniques utilize stretching, gentle pressure, and resistance to help balance the body's nervous, circulatory, and lymphatic systems—thereby contributing to overall health. Some osteopaths also use very gentle movements of your skull and the bone at the bottom of the spine (sacrum). This is a form of treatment called cranial osteopathy or craniosacral therapy.

Osteopathic manipulative treatment has been shown to heal strains and sprains and increase mobility. It also relieves pain[288]—particularly back or neck pain[289] and menstrual pain—and reduces anxiety, depression, tension,[290] and tension-type headaches.[291]

It's also been shown to help everything from asthma, sinus disorders, and pneumonia[292] to carpal tunnel syndrome, sciatica, scoliosis, and osteoarthritis. Even stomach ulcers, irritable bowel syndrome, Parkinson's disease, and high blood pressure have all benefitted from it.

Inflammatory skin diseases also get relief from osteopathic manipulation, which helps promote lymphatic flow, thereby boosting the immune system.[293]

Key Concepts of Osteopathy

To sum up, this is what I and other osteopathic doctors believe:

The body is a unit; each person is a unit of body, mind, and spirit.

The body is capable of self-regulation, self-healing, and health maintenance. When normal adaptability is disrupted, or when environmental changes overcome the body's capacity for self-maintenance, disease may ensue.

Structure and function are reciprocally interrelated. This is the belief that abnormal tissue structure is likely to result in disruptions in tissue function and vice versa.

Treatment is based on understanding the basic principles of body unity, self-regulation, and the interrelationship of structure and function.

Key Facts About Osteopathy

Here is some information [294] about osteopathy that most people don't know:

• **There are currently thirty accredited osteopathic medical schools in the United States** (they're accredited by the American Osteopathic Association Commission on Osteopathic College Accreditation, COCA).

• **The number of DOs in the United States—as of 2014—is more than 92,000**, according to the American Osteopathic Association (AOA).

• **The American Osteopathic College of Dermatology (AOCD) has 431 current board-certified DO dermatologists**, of which I am one.

Healing Movement

Tai chi: This mind/body exercise uses slow, flowing movements that come from Asian martial arts and traditional Chinese medicine. It's said to encourage the flow of qi, the vital energy, that's believed to flow through all living creatures and the universe itself. Its health benefits are backed up in science: numerous studies have shown tai chi to improve health,[295] improve balance,[296] maintain bone density,[297] improve cardiovascular health,[298] increase immunity,[299] and lessen depression and anxiety.[300] More specifically, tai chi has been shown to benefit people with heart failure, fibromyalgia, and osteoarthritis.[301]

Yoga: Most think of yoga as a physical activity, but it was developed in India five thousand years ago as a philosophical religious system to unite the body, mind, and spirit. (The word *yoga* is Sanskrit for "union.") It's intended to improve concentration and meditation by quieting the body and the nervous system or mind. It also increases muscle tone and flexibility and is a powerful stress-management tool that leads to deep relaxation, as well as clear-mindedness, energy, and confidence.[302]

Evidence suggests that regular practice of yoga can help prevent heart disease,[303] carpal tunnel syndrome,[304] asthma,[305] chronic back pain,[306] hypertension,[307] menopausal symptoms like insomnia,[308] arthritis,[309] diabetes,[310] insomnia,[311] thyroid disorders,[312] and digestive disorders like irritable bowel syndrome (IBS).[313]

Mind/Body Approaches

These methods are based on the idea that your thoughts, attitudes, beliefs, and emotions can influence your physical well-being. They use the power of the mind to help improve healing and health. These therapies have been shown to improve the quality of life for people with acute and chronic illness, anxiety, depression, and stress.

Biofeedback or neurofeedback: This noninvasive therapy teaches you to influence your autonomic nervous system—the part of the body that controls involuntary functions like blood pressure, heart rate, muscle tension, and brainwave frequency. It uses electronic equipment to measure biological functions in real time and then reports this information back so you can learn to regulate these functions, which are not normally under conscious control. It can be used to help lower heart rate, blood pressure, or skin temperature and to help you relax more easily.

Brainwave (or EEG) biofeedback or neurofeedback is a special form of biofeedback by which brainwaves—in different parts of the brain—are detected and measured via harmless, noninvasive sensors placed on the scalp. (Specific brain waves need to be firing either with more power or with less in different lobes of the brain to maintain equilibrium.) With the help of a trained practitioner, neurofeedback (also called neurotherapy) is used to help regulate the power of different brain waves, such as alpha waves, which are associated with alert relaxation—often without conscious effort by the patient. Doing so helps restore "balance" in the brain.

Biofeedback has been used to help treat conditions like asthma,[314] irritable bowel syndrome,[315] migraine headaches,[316] epilepsy,[317] hot flashes,[318] insomnia,[319] chronic pain,[320] Raynaud's disease,[321] cardiac arrhythmias,[322] some types of ulcers,[323] anxiety and stress,[324] and nausea associated with chemotherapy.[325] It has been shown to affect levels of the stress hormone cortisol, which can then stabilize insulin levels and lower blood sugar.[326]

The Relaxing Breath

1) Gently move the tip of your tongue against the roof of your mouth, just behind your upper front teeth, and inhale deeply to a mental count of 4. Try to inhale from your stomach area (your diaphragm), not your chest.

2) Hold your breath for a count of 7.

3) Exhale quietly and completely through your mouth with slightly pursed lips to a count of 8.

4) This is one breath cycle. Repeat this cycle for 5 minutes.

Breath work: Breathing is the only function of the body that we perform both voluntarily and involuntarily. Controlling the breath is a powerful technique—also called pranayama—that's a major component of yoga and critical to good health. (*Prana* is the Sanskrit word for breath, spirit, or universal energy.) Through it, we can regulate heart rate, blood pressure, circulation, digestion, and anxiety. It can help improve sleep and energy levels and is an effective stress-management tool. Not only can it help physical and emotional health, it can also be used for mindfulness and spiritual awareness.

I recommend that my patients practice this relaxing breathing meditation for five to ten minutes, one to three times each day. You should try it, too. To do it, make your breathing slow, deep, quiet, and regular. Breathe in through your nose and out through your mouth. This can be done in an office, at a red light, or even waiting in line at a store.

Visualization or guided imagery: What you are thinking about and focusing on can manifest in your life. This is the basis of visualization and guided imagery, a meditation technique where you close your eyes and use your imagination to create peaceful, relaxing visual images in your mind, a goal or a dream. You can add detail to your image like color, sound, motion, and smell. You can even add a song or music. (To engage all the senses, soft music can be playing, a candle can be lit, and aromatherapy scents can be surrounding you.) You can do this while doing your daily breathing exercises and relaxing. The idea behind visualization exercises like this is you can use them to help achieve the life you want.

Often, visualization is guided—meaning someone (in a relaxation, meditation, or yoga class or via an app or digital recording) helps "guide" the images you can picture in your mind.

The idea behind visualization is to engage all the senses to make a connection between the brain and the involuntary nervous system. When the brain's visual cortex is activated—without having direct input from the eyes—it can influence both physical and emotional states, promoting relaxation and healing. Often the best time to use imagery is just before falling asleep and just after waking up, when your imagery can pass more easily into the unconscious mind.

When visualizing, I like to use the words "I am" with what I want to manifest into physical reality. You can use these daily too. For example: "I am healthy," "I am beautiful," "I am confident," "I am strong," "I am intelligent," "I am successful," "I am wealthy," "I am creative," and "I am loving."

Explore not just what you want but also what you are or who you want to be. Put as much detail into the visualization as possible. Think about how you feel when you have what it is you want to manifest. Think about how it looks and feels in your hands. Envision it in detail. You are able to attract into your life all that you desire.

Here are two of my favorite visualizations, taught to me by Rev. Joseph Shiel in Lily Dale, New York:

– **Manifesting visualization** Sit still in a quiet place. Breath normally or simply and gently. Breathe in through the nose and out through pursed lips. Breathe with intention.

Focus on something that means something to you. It could be a sound ("Ahhh" for awakening of the day or light or "Om" for sleep or rest), a picture, a statue, or your breath.

Envision breathing in everything that you want and breathing out anything that is not holding your peace or hurting you. Breathe out the bad memories or the hurt. Take in what you need and breathe out what is not serving your soul well.

Envision that you're breathing it out to the earth. The earth will process it, change it, and bring it back as beauty.

To remind yourself of this process, surround yourself with nature's beauty every day (e.g., a plant or cut flowers). Picture what you want.

You can do this anywhere, anytime. Get yourself intentionally trying to improve and see what you want to see in your life. Everything that you want also wants you. Bring what you want in the universe to yourself. Act as if it is already there, and think of it all the time. Continually improve upon the idea. Refine it. Manifest it. Most importantly, keep it a secret. Then others' negative energies or doubts won't interrupt your goals.

– **Cleansing and healing visualization** Picture yourself sitting quietly, and practice your breathing. Press your tongue against the top palate of your mouth and breath in through your nose and out through your mouth.

Picture a hunter-green liquid soap—and that you have a scrub sponge in each hand. Take your left hand and move clockwise and your right hand and move counterclockwise, and scrub your entire self from head to toe with the scrub sponge and the green liquid. Picture each of your body parts inside and outside—and scrub away any areas that are injured or in need of extra care.

If you feel like you're getting stuck in any one spot, stay in that spot and continue to scrub until it feels good again. Then let all the unhealthy cells and green drain away. Release it into the ground. Then picture a bright white light and scrub with it top to bottom, inside and out again. Then let the white drain out of your feet into Mother Earth.

Water what you just fertilized. Finish by sitting in a moment of gratitude for your life, your gifts, and your challenges. You are being sculpted and molded into the person you are supposed to be. Your soul harbors something special. There is significance to your life.

– **Health benefits of visualization** Visualization has been shown to lower blood pressure,[327] improve insomnia,[328] reduce anxiety and depression,[329] help irritable bowel syndrome (IBS),[330] and help control asthma.[331] Research has shown that it can also help reduce nausea associated with chemotherapy.[332] What's more, visualization has been shown to help encourage a patients' self-healing processes and give them a greater sense of autonomy in relation to a disease and its management.[333]

How to Use Visualization for Relaxation

Sit or lie down in a quiet place. Close your eyes. Take deep, regular, quiet breaths. Then begin to visualize yourself in a beautiful place—real or imagined. For example, imagine that you're in a grassy field with a clear sky overhead. Make it as real as possible by including sounds, smells, colors, and touch. You can focus on the breath—but don't make any attempt to control the breath.

Focus for about five minutes.

Though there is no scientific research on it, some experts also believe you can help your body heal wounds[334] and fight disease by visualizing the anatomy or symptoms of the disease and how they are being fixed or corrected (e.g., if you're undergoing cancer therapy, imagine your immune cells fighting the cancer cells or the chemotherapy helping eliminate the cancer cells).

Taking time to focus on your body and its powerful ability to heal itself can't hurt; at the least, it will relax you—which many studies *have* shown is effective at boosting the immune system. I have had patients tell me firsthand that they have practiced this and believe that, in doing so, they've contributed to curing themselves of their cancer.

Meditation: I've talked a lot about meditation already, but I wanted to give a brief, more formal description of it here. Meditation is the practice by which you can clear your mind by training it to concentrate and cut out all distractions. Essentially, it's a practice by which you can stop the constant inner chatter. It's a way by which you can remember that you're not the voice of your mind—you're merely the one who hears it, day in and day out. Reminding yourself of this helps you connect to your true inner self, and in the process, let go of worry, anxiety, and fear—all of which stoke the fires of unhealthy stress.

Your inner voice can be a source of worry, insecurity, negativity, and anger. Through meditation, you can separate yourself from this and find peace and contentment. You can objectively watch your problems instead of being lost in them. It's easier to deal with a problem if you can handle your reaction to it—without anger, anxiety, or fear.

The first step of meditation is watching or being aware of the constant chatter in your head. This is centered consciousness or focused awareness. When you're centered, you're aware of being conscious. This is true meditation, being able to focus your consciousness completely on one object and also incorporating awareness. And then, slowly you begin to separate the unhealthy chatter from reality. This is a skill that will help you through many situations in life—and one that can bring peace and a true state of health and beauty.

Simple Steps: How to Meditate

Choose a quiet place where you won't be interrupted. Find a comfortable place to sit or lie down.

Focus. While meditating, if your mind begins to wander, bring it back to your breath or your chosen visual object or mantra, without judgment. Just keep practicing this: as your mind wanders, bring it back. When it wanders again, bring it back again.

Try to meditate 5 minutes a day. Then slowly work up to 15 to 30 minutes once or twice a day. If you can't fit in a complete session, try to fit in a few minutes.

If you can, set a meditation timer. This can be a relaxing chime or Tibetan singing bowls; you can find these on your Smartphone (but be sure to shut off your ringer so you're not interrupted). This way, you won't have to be constantly looking at the clock to figure out how much longer you have to meditate. One I like is the free Insight Meditation Timer in the iTunes app store.

The more you practice meditation, the more in control your mind will be—not wandering off in all different thought directions (as we're all prone to doing—thanks to our superbusy lives). The result: the greater awareness you'll have of your body and the world around you (hence, a more relaxed you).

There are many different types of meditation, but all involve directing awareness inward by focusing on an object in the mind's eye, your breath, or a phrase or word (mantra) silently repeated. You can also focus on the heart area while inhaling and exhaling—a technique called heart-centered meditation that helps release fears and sadness, "healing" the heart.

You can practice meditation by sitting in a chair or on the floor, by lying down, or even by walking slowly and mindfully. There's even running meditation, horseback-riding meditation, and kayaking meditation—all based on the idea that you can be mindful of the moment, cutting out all other distractions, in an effort to relax you and clear the mind.

Many meditation proponents believe that meditation stimulates transformative power in the brain and provides you with great conviction and strength to change the course of your life. I believe this could be true, because there's just so much incredible research to date proving the benefits of meditation:

- **Meditation protects the brain.** One University of Oregon study showed, in fact, that meditation can physically change the brain[335,336]—and could even have protective effects against mental illness. The researchers found that after two weeks of practicing meditation, study participants had an increase in the number of signaling connections in the brain, called axonal density. And after a month of practicing regular meditation (about eleven hours of meditation overall), there were even more increases in signaling connections as well as an increase in the protective tissue (called myelin). Study participants also reported better moods overall.

- **Meditation keeps the brain young.** Another fascinating study found that regular meditation can actually stem the tide of age-related brain deterioration or atrophy.[337] These researchers from UCLA found that meditating preserves the brain's gray matter, the tissue that contains the neurons. Pretty powerful stuff!

• **Meditation boosts memory—and more.** Meditation is good for the brain: it can help improve memory, empathy, stress, and sense of self, according to one study from the Massachusetts General Hospital.[338]

• **Meditation can make you happier.** Then there are the studies involving the brainwaves of meditating monks; they show that the actual brain circuitry in long-time meditators is different from that of nonmeditators.[339] When you're upset, anxious, or depressed, the portion of the brain called the amygdala and the right prefrontal cortex become active. When you're in a positive mood, these areas quiet down, and the left prefrontal cortex—an area associated with happiness—becomes more active. Meditating monks appear to have high activity in this "quiet" area—definitely not a random coincidence!

• **Meditation can protect against illness and disease.** Other studies have shown that meditation can decrease heart and respiratory rates and reduce your risk of heart attack and stroke,[340] increase blood flow to the brain,[341] and decrease chronic pain.[342] It's also been shown to treat anxiety disorders,[343] fibromyalgia,[344] irritable bowel syndrome,[345] and PMS.[346]

• **Meditation can reduce pain.** Researchers at Wake Forest School of Medicine found that meditation can actually alter brain activity patterns associated with pain.[347] They found that when a person who is experiencing pain meditates regularly, the pain intensity drops 27 percent—along with a 44 percent drop in emotional pain.

• **Meditation can reduce depression.** Additional research has shown that people who previously were depressed who regularly practice mindfulness-based stress reduction are 50 percent less likely than others to have their depression return.[348] Another study, conducted with veterans who had post-traumatic stress disorder (PTSD), found that after just four sessions of mindfulness-based stress reduction, levels of the primary stress hormone, cortisol, dropped dramatically.[349]

Mindfulness meditation teaches us to alter our response to stress, influencing serotonin production, which regulates mood, sleep, and appetite. Reducing stress also impacts the skin, giving you glowing skin that seems to radiate health from the inside out.

I myself practice this and find it to be relaxing and mind clearing, contributing to a feeling of inner peace. I even believe it has helped me get over colds faster.

So if you don't meditate yet, this might be the time to start. Most experts recommend starting for just five to seven minutes; there are plenty of apps and free guided meditations (I like UCLA Mindful Awareness Center's free guided meditations; you can find them at marc.ucla.edu) that can help you learn how to quiet your mind.

Mindfulness: Mindfulness is a Buddhist technique that brings all of our awareness to the here and now; it's the most popular form of meditation in the Western world. It's about being present—letting your mind run and accepting whatever thoughts come up, while practicing detachment from each thought. Mindfulness is often taught with awareness of the breath.

Progressive muscle relaxation: This relaxation technique involves gently and consciously tightening one muscle at a time, followed by a release of this tension. You can perform it sitting or lying down.

You move either head to toe or toe to head with each muscle group, paying attention to how your body feels as you squeeze and release. When you finish, you feel relaxed from head to toe.

To do it: Close your eyes and focus, first, on the gentle rhythm of your breathing (but don't try to control your breath). Then focus on a single muscle group, and while taking a deep breath, tense all the muscles in that area for around five seconds. Slowly relax the area as you exhale and let the stress flow from your body. Move down or up the body. Practice this for ten to fifteen minutes each day. If you have a busy day with little time for yourself, perform an abbreviated version for a few minutes on the area of your body where you hold most of your tension (often, the neck and shoulders for many people).

Progressive muscle relaxation can help those with anxiety,[350] asthma,[351] insomnia,[352] high blood pressure,[353] and chronic pain.[354]

Don't Love to Meditate? Consider This

If you've tried meditation and just don't love it, you may be doing the wrong kind of meditation for you. In fact, when it comes to meditation, one size (or kind of meditation) definitely does *not* fit all. That's the conclusion of researchers from the San Francisco State University Institute for Holistic Health Studies.[355] Their research suggests that picking the method of meditation you like—not what happens to be the latest trend—will help you stick with it for the long haul. Here's a guide:

Transcendental meditation: During this meditation, you sit with your eyes closed and your back straight (ideally in the lotus or half-lotus position) while focusing on—and repeating—a sound or mantra.

Guided visualization: This meditation involves focusing your attention on imaginary visual images and can often be done listening to a speaker (either live or via a recording).

Chakra meditation: Using specific visualizations about the major chakras (or energy centers in the body), you visualize opening and cleansing these "areas" of the body. This is typically used when an area of your body is unhealthy—why it's also called "healing meditation."

Mindfulness mediation: During this meditation, you focus on the breath—in and out—while practice being present in the moment without letting your mind fill up with thoughts.

Practice Mindful Meditation—While you Eat

So many of us rush through our meals, often eating in front of the TV, a computer at our desk, or in the car. Eating slowly and mindfully will result in better digestion—and possibly even weight loss: the more mindful you are, the more satisfied you'll be—and the less food you'll be "hungry" for later on.

To practice mindfulness while you're eating:

1) Hold a piece of fruit (like a grape) or a piece of popcorn in your hand. Think about how it looks. What is the color, size, and shape? Next think about how it feels. Is it heavy, light, smooth, or rough? What does it smell like?

2) Place it in your mouth without chewing and think about how it feels. Texture? Now chew it slowly. How does it feel and taste?

3) Focus on all of these aspects as you chew and swallow. Once you've done this, try eating an entire meal with focus on how each bite feels and tastes in your mouth—and you will be on your way to eating mindfully.

Healing Therapies

Animal-assisted therapy: There's incredible evidence—firsthand and in clinical research—that there's an emotional bond between people and animals that can have benefits on emotional and physical health. This is the philosophy behind animal therapy, which has been formally used since the 1940s when an army corporal brought his Yorkshire terrier to a hospital to cheer wounded shoulders.

Animal therapy uses interaction with trained animals—from dogs and cats to horses and even dolphins—to enhance physical, emotional, and social well-being; improve self-esteem; and reduce anxiety. I myself have two Yorkies and know firsthand their comforting effects!

Research shows that animals can help with anxiety, depression, and social isolation,[356] and can lower blood pressure and cholesterol.[357] It's also been shown—particularly with therapy dogs—to help the emotional well-being of some cancer patients.[358]

Studies have shown that people with pets, namely dogs, have less of something called "cardiovascular reactivity" when stressed.[359] This means that when pet owners are stressed, their heart rate and blood pressure rise and return to normal more quickly. Researchers attribute this to a decrease in cortisol levels because of owning a pet.

Animal therapy has also been used to help people with conditions like cerebral palsy;[360] autism, ADHD, and dyslexia;[361] and Down syndrome.[362] Plus, it's shown to be effective at calming children who have experienced physical or emotional trauma. (A good website that offers more information on this is petpartners.org.)

Aromatherapy: Aromatic plants have been used in healing for millennia, and essential oils have been used since the Middle Ages. Modern aromatherapy was founded—and the term coined—in the 1920s by French chemist Rene-Maurice Gattefosse. After burning his hand in a lab explosion, he put the burned skin in a bowl of lavender oil and was surprised to find that his burns healed quickly—without infection, pain, or scarring. He then started investigating essential oils in treating various skin conditions. He studied oils from flowers, leaves, fruits, barks, and roots and how they affected physical and mental health.

In France and Japan, medical aromatherapy is an established and accepted field. The theory behind it: physiologic responses develop via scent receptors in the nose that send chemical messages through nerves to the brain. (One study found that the skin contains olfactory receptors.[363]) This is believed to trigger emotional and physiological effects that can influence the immune, circulatory, and respiratory systems.

Aromatherapy has been shown to reduce pain and anxiety.[364] But since each essential oil has hundreds of natural chemical parts, the benefits of aromatherapy are extensive. Certain natural chemicals called aldehydes in lemon balm, for example, have been studied for their ability to reduce inflammation.[365] Other research has shown that lemon oil improves mood.[366] Natural chemicals, called ketones, in rosemary and eucalyptus seem to help reduce mucus production.[367] Grapefruit oil appears to stimulate the brain to produce natural painkillers, enkephalins (one type of endorphins).[368]

But don't apply essential oils directly on the skin; I've seen patients with allergic contact dermatitis that has developed from placing essential oils directly on the skin. Instead, inhale essential oils in a room diffuser, place drops nearby (e.g., on a pillowcase or eye mask), or breathe them from an individual inhaler.

Art therapy: Research shows that positive imagery can benefit patients in various areas of health care—which is why many health-care centers and hospitals are putting more thought into what they showcase on their walls and in their patient areas. These health-care centers are also offering art-therapy classes as a way for patients and their families to express what they're going through in a different way. This type of therapy is often used by cancer patients, pediatric patients, and those who have experienced physical or emotional trauma.

Research shows, for example, that calming, peaceful artwork in hospitals can help encourage a patient's healing process, while the opposite—stark, depressing walls and even the wrong kind of art, like disturbing art—can cause physical distress and even hinder healing. One review of research, published in the *American Journal of Public Health*, found that visual art helps "express experiences, such as a diagnosis of cancer, that are too difficult to put into words" and can be a "refuge from the intense emotions associated with illness."[369]

There is also some evidence that art can help reduce hospital stays: in studies of both cancer and cardiovascular patients, those who had access to art (for example, a picture of a stress-relieving landscape on their wall) were better able to self-manage chronic pain (and had a decreased need for narcotic pain medication)[370] and checked out of the hospital earlier than those who didn't have access to the healing art.[371]

Additional research shows that art can help with quality of life for those suffering from Alzheimer's disease.[372]

But you don't need to be suffering from disease or be in a hospital to appreciate or reap the health benefits of art. A University of California, Berkeley study found that that taking in art, nature, and even religion (e.g., visiting museums or religious sites or being out in nature)—which inspire positive emotions like awe and wonder—may be enough make people act kinder and more altruistically.[373] Awe, say the researchers, makes people realize that life is bigger than them and causes them to want to act selflessly. What's more, these feelings of awe and wonder also lower levels of proinflammatory cytokines. Sustained high levels of cytokines are associated with poor health and disorders such as type 2 diabetes, heart disease, arthritis, depression, and Alzheimer's.

Healing Touch: Healing Touch is a therapy that helps restore and balance energy in the body. It was founded in 1989 by Janet Mentgen, a registered nurse. Practitioners use their hands and very light or near-the-body touch to promote relaxation and balance the energy that surrounds the body. The goal is to remove energetic blockages (similar to acupuncture or acupressure, which removes energy blockages to facilitate the flow of qi, to facilitate healing). There are various types of this approach, including Reiki, Energy Field Therapy, and Therapeutic Touch.

The practitioner focuses on areas where the energy field is felt to be stagnant or not flowing or on the seven main energy centers called chakras in yoga philosophy. (*Chakra* is a Sanskrit term for energy centers that are believed to connect the physical and energetic body.) Some people have referred to these chakras as our own invisible, rechargeable batteries that connect our spiritual bodies to our physical ones.

The 7 Chakras

The 7 chakras work together to balance the body—and spirit. When any one chakra is blocked, it can trigger emotional and health problems.

1) Root Chakra (at the base of the spine) represents our foundation and plays a part in us feeling (or not feeling) grounded. It's the chakra closest to the earth. Feelings of fear usually signal a blockage in this chakra.

2) Sacral Chakra (in lower abdomen) rules our sense of abundance and wellbeing, as well as pleasure and sexuality. Emotional problems usually indicate a blockage in this chakra.

3) Solar Plexus Chakra (in the upper abdomen) represents our ability to be self-confident and in control. Anger and lack of direction are usually signs of a blockage in this chakra.

4) Heart Chakra (in the chest) rules love. Lack of compassion and inhumanity usually manifest when this chakra is blocked.

5) Throat Chakra (in the throat) governs our ability to express ourselves. Creative blocks and inability to communicate usually indicate problems with this chakra.

6) Third-Eye Chakra (between the brows) rules imagination, intuition, and wisdom. Lack of foresight, mental rigidity, and even depression usually signify a blockage in this chakra.

7) Crown Chakra (on the top of the head) governs inner and outer beauty and our spirituality. Psychological problems usually signal a blockage of this chakra.

Reiki: Reiki means universal life energy and was developed in Japan by Mikao Usui, who was inspired to devise a system of spiritual development—not a religion—that would be accessible to all people. He wanted a holistic system that could take the follower on a path to enlightenment without the constraints of organized religion.

One of Usui's most famous quotes explains the essence of Reiki:

> *"The Universe is me, and I am the Universe. The Universe exists in me, and I exist in the Universe. Light exists in me, and I exist in the light."*

I recently had the opportunity to have a Reiki healing done on me in Lily Dale, New York (the largest spiritual community and library in the world). It's there that I discovered that Reiki is one of the tools we can use to guide us through life. It promotes physical health, mental clarity, and spiritual advancement—and can be incorporated into any lifestyle.[374]

The five elements of Reiki are:

(1) The five spiritual principles or precepts: These are to be recited daily, to be followed throughout the day, or to be meditated on:

Do not anger.
Do not worry.
Be humble.
Be honest in your work.
Be compassionate to yourself and others.

(2) Breathing techniques: As I've mentioned earlier, breathing is so important to health and wellness. This includes diaphragmatic breathing and mindfulness breathing.

(3) Hands-on palm healing: We all use our hands to heal, such as when we touch people to hug or reassure them. We all give the comfort of touch. Reiki or palm healing, as it translates from the Japanese word *Tenohira,* is a system of transmitting healing energy to oneself or others.

(4) Symbols and mantras: A mantra, as I've mentioned earlier, is a word or sound that's repeated as a form of meditation.

(5) Attunements: An attunement is a form of spiritual empowerment that passes through the teacher to the student, activating the ability to draw in more energy based on individual need. This enables them to become more effective channels for the Reiki energy.

Reiki healers say they can feel the blocks in your energy and help you rebalance your energy. I didn't feel anything during the actual healing I had done, but I did feel good overall immediately afterward—a feeling that lasted for weeks.

Common uses include headaches, anxiety, and insomnia. Many say the treatment produces a state of deep calm and relaxation. Research has shown that Healing Touch can also help with wound healing and decreased pain[375]—which is why many hospitals are incorporating it into their surgery centers and cancer departments.

Herbal medicine: Herbal medicine relies on plants or plant extracts—which are rich in a variety of natural chemical compounds—as treatments. It's been used since ancient times in many different cultures throughout the world as way of keeping the body healthy and treating illness.

When we use cooking herbs and spices that have disease-preventing effects, for example, we're taking advantage of herbal health benefits. Look for herbal preparations that have been cultivated organically and only from reputable sources (which stand by their ingredients and the potency of the herbs).

Here are some of the top health-promoting herbs:

Aloe reduces redness and swelling from burns and skin inflammation; it also calms skin.

Arnica helps reduce bruising and swelling.

Basil is an anti-inflammatory and antibacterial that may also fight viruses.

Cilantro and coriander are natural preservatives and antibacterials that aid in detoxification.

Cinnamon is an antifungal that also may improve glucose and lipids in patients with diabetes.[376] Cinnamaldehyde—the compound that gives cinnamon its distinctive flavor and smell—has also been shown to help prevent cancer.[377]

Dill is an antibacterial that aids in digestion, and it is a breath freshener.

Garlic is a powerful anti-inflammatory and immune booster.

Ginger helps aid indigestion and nausea.

Mint is a natural decongestant that also soothes indigestion and calms and cools the skin (from insect bites, rashes, and other irritations).

Oregano is a powerful antibacterial and anti-inflammatory that may also slow the progression of cancer.[378]

Parsley supports kidney function (and natural detoxification), is an anti-inflammatory, and may inhibit the development of cancer.[379]

Rosemary is a potent anti-inflammatory, reduces the formation of cancer-causing agents during cooking, and may help keep eyesight sharp.[380]

Thyme is an antimicrobial and antibacterial that helps treat acne and skin fungal infections, protects against foodborne infections,[381] and protects against cancer.[382]

Turmeric or curcumin is a powerful inflammatory, protects against cancer,[383] and may boost memory[384] and protect against Alzheimer's disease.[385]

Music therapy: Music has the power to make us feel better. Most of us know this intuitively, as listening to our favorite tunes just makes us feel happier. But science is discovering that it can help do more than just boost our mood: music also seems to help reduce pain and anxiety, particularly in patients undergoing surgery.

One study used soothing music with patients undergoing thoracic surgery; it found that listening to just thirty minutes of soft music a day for three days helped these patients experience less postoperative pain and anxiety.[386] Not to mention, these patients also had lower blood pressure and heart rate. This study finding was backed up by other research, which found that patients who listen to music before, during, and after surgery had overall less pain and anxiety—and had less need for pain medication.[387] Another study found that music could help reduce pain from conditions like fibromyalgia.[388]

What's more, researchers are also finding that when surgeons listen to their preferred music during surgery, they take less time to close surgical wounds—and the quality of these surgical closures improve, too.[389]

None of this surprises me, though. The power of music was something that I discovered firsthand way back when I was in junior high. My science-class assignment was to write and perform an at-home experiment that could be measured somehow. I remember cooking with my grandmother on the Saturday afternoon after I was given my homework and thinking about what I wanted to measure. I knew that I had to keep it within a low budget, but I also wanted an A.

My grandmother and I were making an avocado salad at the time, and it hit me: I would measure whether an avocado plant would grow any differently if exposed or not exposed to music. (I loved listening to music then—and still do today—and intuitively, even at that young age, I knew that music would probably make a difference in a plant's growth.) My grandmother gave me two pits from the avocados we were using for our salad, and I soaked them in water so they could take root.

Before long, I was planting them in soil. I positioned both plants in front of a window, on the same side of the house but in different rooms. One plant had constant low-level music playing next to it, and the other didn't. I then spent the next several weeks watering them with the same amount of water, carefully measuring their growth, and charting my results. As expected, the plant that was exposed to music grew significantly larger. (And yes, I did get an A on the assignment, which made me so happy and proud—and planted the seeds for a career in holistic health and wellness!)

Nature therapy: Plenty of research shows that being outdoors—with its fresh air, trees, and elements of nature including birds and wildlife—helps relax us and keep us healthy by reducing blood pressure, heart rate, muscle tension, and stress.

In fact, Japanese researchers have shown that spending a short time in nature actually boosts the activity of immune cells—which help fight illness and disease—for up to seven days.[390] Other researchers have shown that walking outdoors among trees and wildlife boosts energy[391] as well as creativity.[392]

Numerous studies have shown the stress-reducing benefits of being surrounded by nature. One study, conducted at Stanford University, found that walking for just ninety minutes in nature actually reduced activity in an area of the brain (the subgenual prefrontal cortex) associated with anxiety and depression.[393] Another study found that taking regular "micro breaks" (forty-second breaks) throughout the day to look at nature—or even pictures of nature—helps reduce stress and mental fatigue.[394]

Nature can also boost a patient's recovery and reduce pain: one study conducted at Texas A&M University found that patients who had a view of trees outside their hospital rooms actually healed faster and had less pain than those patients whose windows looked out at a wall.[395]

Whole-Body Healing Systems

Ayurvedic medicine: This healing system originated in northern India over five thousand years ago. The word *ayurveda* is a Sanskrit term that means the science of life or life knowledge. Its guiding principle is that the mind and body are inseparable, a whole-body approach that incorporates meditation, herbalism, a balanced diet that includes the six ayurvedic tastes (sweet, salty, sour, pungent, bitter, and astringent), yoga, bodywork, detoxification, healthy relationships, and stress management (including meditation) to promote health. It defines health as a state of energy that balances all aspects of life: sleep, diet, physical activity, plant and mineral remedies, and sexual activity.

In fact, in ayurveda, this whole-body balanced approach to health is revealed in how you look. Pure beauty, according to ayurveda, is clear, glowing skin; silky hair; happy eyes; youthfulness; and even a pleasant smell. This is the result of inner and outer happiness and health (including a strengthened immune system) that ayurveda sums up as something called ojas (a Sanskrit word pronounced *oh-jus*). Ojas is referred to in ayurveda as the sap of life.

Traditional Chinese medicine: This healing system developed in China more than two thousand years ago. It considers how the human body interacts with all aspects of life and the environment, like ayurvedic medicine. It teaches that the balance of health depends on the unobstructed flow of life energy, or qi, through the body along meridian pathways.

Practitioners believe that disease is the result of disruptions in the circulation of qi. This is why therapies are directed at helping balance and improve the flow of qi, through herbal medicine, acupuncture, acupressure, martial arts, and energy techniques like qi gong. (Qi gong integrates posture, body movements, breathing, and focused intention to help improve mental and physical health.)

Everyday Enlightenment

Chronic stress can result in a disconnected body, mind, and spirit. But these parts need to be in sync for true health and beauty. This is something that I believe in wholeheartedly.

In the words of the Greek philosopher Plato:

> *"The cure of the part should not be attempted without treatment of the whole. No attempt should be made to cure the body without the soul...This is the error of our day, that physicians first separate the soul from the body."*

This is why, whenever my patients come into my office, I offer them much more than just skin-care advice. I talk to them about their lives, too, and as a result, they tell me they leave feeling better about themselves. I'm a big believer that confidence and happiness in one's life—along with strong self-esteem—contributes to great skin and a healthy body as well.

Here's the key: what I've found is that it's often the simplest gestures every day that can make us feel better, boost our mood, and calm us—reducing stress and boosting health, including the health of our skin. I call this everyday spiritual enlightenment. Here are a few of the simple reminders that I give to my patients; these are good bits of advice for everyone:

✓ **Go out and enjoy life; don't wait for the right moment.** How many of us wait for enough money or the exact right time to take a vacation or do something that we love? So many unused vacation days go to waste for so many Americans. Don't wait: schedule that time off or visit that place you've always wanted to see. Live each day to its fullest and appreciate the time you've been given.

✓ **Decide to be happy.** We all have an underlying pattern of thoughts that plays over and over in our minds. Become aware of them and direct them in a more positive way (this becomes easier once you spend time in quiet thought or meditation). Things will happen that challenge you, but decide to keep a good attitude regardless of what happens. In fact, just trying to be happy has been shown in studies to make you more positive overall.[396] And as Lao Tzu has said:

"If you correct your mind, the rest of your life will fall into place."

Being happy is the true spiritual path. Any tests that come along (and there will be many!) will offer you opportunity for spiritual growth. Remember: there is no growth without difficulty. Your life is meant to be enjoyed and appreciated, and experiences are to be learned from. Experiences, though, should not determine our happiness. You determine if you're happy. Enjoy the life that comes at you. If you think about the last thing that bothered you and what happened when you let it ruin your day, you realize that you had no benefit from the ruined day. We all have limited time left in our lives, and it should be enjoyed and spent being happy.

✓ **Be accepting of others**. The world would be a very boring place if we all were exactly the same physically and all had the same personality. We should be accepting of each other's differences, because it is these differences that make our world the amazing place that it is. Variety is the spice of life. Through acceptance you can achieve inner peace.

✓ **Don't just evaluate situations with your mind;** pay attention to how you feel (your gut response or intuition), too, and act on them. Your mind can lie, but your feelings and emotions won't. They are aligning you with your true path, your inner self. I liken the gut to our own inner GPS.

It is Albert Einstein who once said:

> *"The intuitive mind is a sacred gift and the rational mind is a faithful servant. We have created a society that honors the servant and has forgotten the gift."*

How true! Follow your dreams or inner thoughts and desires. Follow the calling you feel deep within you.

✓ **Cultivate your spiritual side.** Set aside time every day to connect to your higher self with moments of silence.

✓ **Go with the flow.** Life throws both pleasant and unpleasant things our way. I've learned that life is easier if you accept the things that happen for what they are and move on. Try not to hold on to the negative, but let it pass by or through. Try not to hold too tightly even to the good. By holding on to the good, you're living in the past. Try to live and appreciate each moment for what it is.

When bad happens, know that it's an opportunity for growth. It may not be easy, and you may not enjoy it, but you're able to learn and grow from the bad—and just know that something good will come in the end.

Think of yourself standing in the middle of a shallow moving river. You're there to experience the river or life but not to try to stop it or control the flow. Life will be less stressful if you're accepting of it. Another way to envision it is this: See yourself in a car driving down the road of life. Watch the trees, cars, and homes pass by, but keep yourself in the moment and don't think about what you previously saw.

In the words of George Orwell:

"Happiness can only exist in acceptance."

Enjoy life; accept what happens and the things that you cannot change. Don't try to resist or fight it—and you'll find that you're more peaceful and more resilient with anything life sends your way.

✓ **Live in the now, not in the yesterday or tomorrow.** Enjoy and feel the power of the moment. Be there totally. Life is now. Feel your presence. Albert Einstein spoke these words:

"I never think of the future; it comes soon enough."

I also love this from the Dalai Lama:

"The Dalai Lama, when asked what surprised him most about humanity, answered, 'Man. Because he sacrifices his health in order to make money. Then he sacrifices money to recuperate this health. And then he is so anxious about the future that he does not enjoy the present; the result being that he does not live in the present or the future; he lives as if he is never going to die, and then dies having never really lived.'"

✓ **Find something to be thankful for every day.** Be thankful to be alive, for family, for friends, for health, for a good deed from a stranger.

✓ **Learn how to forgive.** Letting go of bitterness and grudges helps free up that energy that you're devoting to the negativity. Forgiveness, research has shown, is also good for your health, bettering your sleep quality, your blood pressure, your heart rate (and your heart health), your anxiety levels, rates of depression, stress, and even cholesterol levels.[397] So do your health a favor: add more peace to your life and forgive!

✓ **Don't only focus on your outer purpose or goal** (career, riches) but also on each step of the way and how you build your inner purpose and consciousness. This follows the philosophy: "Create a life that feels good on the inside, not one that just looks good on the outside."

Our journey in life has both an outer purpose (to reach a goal or accomplish something) and an inner purpose (this is the journey into yourself)—and they're both intricately entwined and both essential to your overall health. In fact, one fascinating study actually found that having a purpose in life motivates people to optimize their health, which means they're more likely to take care of themselves.[398]

✓ **Avoid repetitive negative thoughts**, such as judgment, criticism, hatred, or anger. Try to focus on the positive. In the words of the Dalai Lama:

> *"The ultimate creator is the human mind or consciousness. It immediately creates an atmosphere: sometimes pleasant, sometimes unpleasant. Then this energy, it creates a chain reaction on two levels, one with immediate effect, one with a long-term effect. So you see, in order to change the external thing, we must first change the routine within ourselves."*

✓ **Realize there is good in everything that happens.** In the words of Ram Dass:

> *"Everything in your life is there as a vehicle for transformation. Use it!"*

The things that we learn through our experiences—both good and bad—help better us, make us grow, and even empower us. I love this, too, from Elisabeth Kübler-Ross:[399]

> *"The most beautiful people we have known are those who have known defeat, known suffering, known struggle, known loss, and have found their way out of the depths. These persons have an appreciation, a sensitivity, and an understanding of life that fills them with compassion, gentleness and a deep loving concern. Beautiful people do not just happen.*
>
> *"With time, I have come to understand that both the positive and negative things that come into my life are blessings. I am able to grow through my difficulties and advance spiritually...Spiritual advances that we make in life are largely preceded by difficulty.*
>
> *"I asked a question to one of my spiritual teachers: Why do we have to go through difficulties in our lives, starting in childhood, and he answered me with an analogy of creating a sculpture out of stone. His answer stuck with me and I've been sharing it with everyone since.*
>
> *"The artist must bang away at the stone in order to create a beautiful artistic sculpture or statue. The trauma to the stone equates to our pain in life. The trauma that we receive helps us to become who we are, it shapes us and makes us who we are, a beautiful being. When one of my family is faced with a challenge or difficulty we like to say a quote from the Disney movie,* Meet the Robinsons, *that we have watched together several times. We say, 'Let go of the past and keep moving forward.'"*

So the next time you experience something that you feel is bad, look deeper into it to find the lesson or positive that came from it. It may take some time, but eventually you'll be able to find something positive that you can learn from and even use to help others.

✓ **Be selective of those in your inner circle.** If someone is always negative, complaining, and criticizing others, it will also affect you. Limit your time in bad relationships. Like Mom always used to say, be careful of the friends you choose.

✓ **Show kindness, compassion, and generosity to others.** It's contagious and just feels good! And it may also be hardwired, in our brains, to be giving. Scientists are starting to discover that we have circuits in our brain that regulate empathy and the desire to help others.[400] What's more, the areas of the brain involved give off a pleasurable response—as well as giving off brain chemicals like oxytocin, the hormone that promotes social bonding, and dopamine, the pleasure chemical—once we act on our altruistic impulses.

✓ **Follow your dreams.** I truly believe that if you dream it, you can do it. It's important to believe in yourself, love yourself, and fulfill your innermost dreams—no matter what other people say or who believes in you or not. I wanted to share my own personal stories with you about this.

When I was in my junior year of high school, I had a meeting with my high-school counselor to discuss what I wanted to do after high school. He asked me, "What are your plans after you graduate?" I told him that I wanted to go to college at the University of Michigan, that this was my dream. He told me that I could not go to the University of Michigan because I was a girl and that I was going to "stay home and have babies." (It's crazy now to think that someone would have said this, but this is what some people believed when I was in school.)

I told him that I didn't want to stay home and that my dream was to go to Michigan. He said that he would not fill out a college application with me or release my transcripts and that our meeting was over. I went home and cried. When my mother returned home from work, she asked me why I was crying. I told her what my counselor said. She asked me what I wanted, and I told her. She then told me to follow my dreams and to make it happen. I asked how, and she said, "You'll figure it out." In the end, I applied myself and ended up getting accepted. I followed my dreams, didn't give up, and made it happen!

I had a similar story in medical school. When I was in medical school, I knew that I wanted to be a dermatologist, more than anything. When performing clinical rotations third year, you're given a choice of electives for the first time. For my first elective, I chose a dermatology rotation with a local female dermatologist. While I was with her, she asked me what specialty I wanted to go into. I told her dermatology and how excited I was to be experiencing and learning about it. She then told me that I would never get in, that it was too hard, and to not even bother trying. Even after I explained my passion, straight-A grades, research experience, and awards, she told me I would never make it. I was discouraged, but I didn't give up on my dream. It was a long road, but again, I made it happen!

By following your heart, you're staying aligned with your higher self. Work toward your true path and let the universe take care of the details. I have a distinct inner excitement that cannot be ignored when I listen to my inner self. It's then that I know without a doubt that I must do certain things. Just as I followed through on my dreams, so too can you—no matter what obstacles or negativity you face.

➔**Where do you go from here?** Consider ojas—from ayurvedic medicine—as your ultimate goal. True inner and outer beauty and health that radiates from a relaxed, peaceful state. This state of balance is a result of proper diet and finding ways to manage stress every day, but it's also a result of exercise and sleep. And that's what I want to talk about in the coming chapters: what you need, how to incorporate both into a busy life, and why it's so important to this cultivation of the ojas—for longevity and true inner and outer beauty.

CHAPTER 3

Rethink Your Exercise Strategy

"To enjoy the glow of good health, you must exercise."

~ *Gene Tunney*

We all know that exercise is important for our health. In fact, getting people in the United States to be more active could cut yearly medical costs by more than $70 billion.[401] But it's so hard to translate this knowledge into action. I experience this firsthand, but I've learned to make time for exercise—and you can, too. It's not easy, but it is doable. Despite having a busy dermatology practice and two young (and very active!) children, I've learned to make time for yoga, exercise classes, workout videos (my first one was Jane Fonda in the late '80s!), swimming laps, and walking, because moving my body is essential for me to stay healthy and happy. And believe me, there are plenty of days when I just don't want to exercise because of my busy schedule—but I force myself to do it anyway and end up being incredibly happy I did!

In fact, I always keep exercise videos (including yoga videos) around for those days when I don't have time to drive to the gym—or it's just too cold to go outside, which is often during the winter months. One of my favorites is a quick twenty-five-minute full-body workout; it's perfect for time-crunched days, because it's fast and effective!

It was during medical school that I learned just how important exercise is to overall well-being. I had a treadmill in my apartment, and—despite long, grueling study hours and practical training in the hospital—I made it a point to walk on the treadmill four or five times a week. I tried to do anywhere from thirty minutes to an hour. A few light weights for strength training, regular stretching, and exercise videos helped complete my not-so-fancy apartment routine.

This commitment to exercise—in spite of my busy schedule—made all the difference for me. It cleared my mind so I could process everything better. I felt better; I was less stressed and happier overall. Plus, I had more energy. And I got sick much less than I ever did before, despite having a demanding workload.

The Ikarians and Okinawans also have a commitment to moving every day. And most of the time, this exercise is gardening, walking, or doing yard work—activities that inspire them and motivate them to stay active.

It's no secret that exercise can make a huge difference in how you feel, how often you get sick (it's proven that exercise boosts your immunity), your stress levels, how well you sleep, and how youthful your skin looks. A healthy, radiant glow is common after a heart-pumping workout for good reason: as you boost your circulation, you also boost blood flow—rich in oxygen and nutrients—to the skin. As circulation and sweat increases, so too does the removal of toxins from the body through your pores, which also contributes to your overall health.

Exercise can also boost the body's (and the skin's) antioxidant system. According to research from North Arizona University, just one exercise session has the power to boost the body's antioxidant system and its ability to ward off oxidative stress.[402] So imagine what regular exercise can do for your skin—and your body overall!

I share my own story of exercise with my patients all the time and recommend that every one of my patients get out and move their body. It should be part of everyone's healthy skin—and healthy body—routine.

The most common reason people say they don't exercise is time. (Lack of energy—from lack of sleep; a diet heavy in processed foods, sugar, and caffeine; and long days—is usually a close second.) But I've found that repeating this mantra helps motivate me to get moving when I'm busy:

"I lovingly do everything I can to assist my body in maintaining perfect health."

In this next step, I share some practical techniques to block out time on your schedule for exercise (the way you would an important meeting or event)—and why it's so incredibly important to do so.

Bottom line: our bodies are meant to move—which is why exercise, be it a walk around the block or an intense cardio workout at the gym, can make you feel great. And if you ask, "What's better: cardio or strength training?" I have this to say: both are good for your health, but for different reasons.

Aerobic exercise works the heart, which is a muscle. It also burns calories and fat. But strength training builds muscle, which boosts your bone strength and your resting metabolism, helping you burn more calories while you're sitting. (The more muscle you have, the more calories you'll burn all day long. Also, the more muscle you have, the stronger your bones.)

These are good reasons to consistently include both cardiovascular exercise, or aerobic exercise, and strength training in your routine.

How Much Exercise Is Enough?

This is a question that many people have. I believe that just moving your body as much as you can is helpful. But people often like a "prescription" for exercise, specifically how much they should exercise every day and every week. But this is important: always check with your doctor before engaging in any form of exercise—cardio or strength training—to be sure your body and your heart can handle what you're doing.

I agree with what the researchers recommend. Most of the studies showing the positive effects of exercising on the heart and the health use a guideline of thirty to sixty minutes of continuous exercise three days per week. The intensity is usually 60–75 percent of your max heart rate. (This basically tells you how much you should be exercising based on your age.)

To determine your max heart rate: subtract your age from 220. So if you're forty-five, your maximum heart rate is 175—60 percent of that is a heart rate of 105 beats per minute, and 75 percent is a heart rate of 131 beats per minute. If you're using a heart-rate monitor, it should register between 105 and 131 beats to get heart-healthy benefits.

If you exercise too hard (over your maximum heart rate), you're straining—which is bad for your heart—and you need to slow down. If it's too low, you're not challenging your heart muscle enough to gain real benefits.

Keep in mind, if you can exercise five or even six days a week—taking one day to rest—that's even better for you.[403] But three days a week should be the minimum goal.

Top Ten Reasons to Exercise

(1) It boosts brainpower. Exercise is so powerful it actually causes the creation of new neurons in the brain and, specifically, the hippocampus—the center of learning and memory.[404] (And stress, interestingly, can hamper this growth of new neurons.) But aerobic exercise is what gets this hippocampus-boosting result: resistance training, balance training, and muscle-toning exercises did not get the same results[405] (though these exercises are still good for you—just in other ways). This results in improved alertness and concentration and overall cognitive function.

Exercise also seems to boost the brain by reducing inflammation in the body and in the brain. When you exercise, your fat and muscle tissue release anti-inflammatory cytokines—or proteins that affect the interactions between cells—into your blood, which accounts for this drop in inflammation.[406] This helps keep brain cells healthy.

Researchers even go so far as to say that exercise actually changes the brain for the better, protecting it from age-related memory changes.[407] In essence, exercise keeps the brain young.

(2) It makes you feel great. This is a result of the energy boost and reduction in fatigue you get from working out. You also feel amazing during and after exercise because of the secretion of a finely choreographed symphony of mood-boosting chemicals, or neuropeptides, in the body called endorphins. (These are what give you the so-called runner's high.)

Endorphins are neurotransmitters, or chemicals that pass electrical signals from one neuron to the next in the nervous system. These neurotransmitters—which are secreted from the pituitary gland, the spinal cord, and throughout the brain and nervous system—play a key role in the functioning of the central nervous system. When they're released, as they are after exercise, after massage, and even after eating hot chili peppers, they interact with receptors in brain cells responsible for blocking pain (both physical and mental) and controlling emotion.

They also interact with what are called opiate receptors in the brain, reducing our perception of pain. That's why endorphins have a similar—albeit natural and nonaddictive—effect on the brain as powerful drugs like morphine and codeine, which act on these same opiate receptors. This may be why athletes are able to push through pain to win a game—and why, despite an intense body-challenging workout, we feel almost euphoric.

(3) It keeps your weight in check. Fat cells are able to produce estrogen; the more weight you're carrying, the more estrogen that's circulating in your body—and the higher your risk of diseases like cancer. Excess weight can also increase your risk of diabetes and heart disease.[408]

What's more, as we get older, our body holds on to these estrogen-producing fat cells—making it harder to lose weight without exercise.

(4) It reduces the amount of circulating hormones in the body. In women, exercise reduces the amount of estrogen that's circulating in the body—key to a reduced risk of diseases like breast cancer.[409] (Excess estrogen in the body has been linked to breast cancer.)

(5) It boosts your immunity. Exercise appears to boost the body's response to invading viruses or bacteria, but only if it's moderate exercise (not intense exercise).

Moderate exercise, such as a leisurely jog or walk, as opposed to physically intense exercise (or exercise for a prolonged period of time, usually an hour or more) has been found to be better for the immune system. This is the type of exercise practiced by the Okinawans and Ikarians—further proof that this type of regular exercise contributes to longevity.

Intense workouts—a power run, an intense cycling session, or even running a marathon—have been found to temporarily depress the immune system anywhere from a few hours to a few days, much in the way sugar suppresses the immune system for up to three hours after eating it. In fact, if you do it after you catch a bug, intense exercise can make the symptoms and severity of an illness worse.

Moderate regular exercise, on the other hand, appears to suppress something called TH_1 cells (immune cells that induce inflammation, which is typically the body's first response against an invading virus) and increase TH_2 cells (which produce an anti-inflammatory response). Intense exercise suppresses the TH_1 too much, shutting down this first line of defense before it has time to do what it needs to do.[410]

So get out there and do a moderate workout every day. And if you love an intense exercise every now and then, be sure to balance it out with moderate exercise so your immune system doesn't take a hit.

Simple Strength Training

Some easy ways to add strength training to your routine:

✓ **Wear a walking vest.** These adjustable weighted vests can be worn daily to transform your daily walks into strength-training ones.

✓ **Do bodyweight exercises.** Push-ups are the easiest exercises to do. You need no equipment and can do them anywhere. Other good options include squats (for your legs) and crunches (for your abs).

✓ **Try using resistance tubing.** These stretchy, lightweight pieces of latex provide resistance (and strength training) when stretched. (Tip: the lighter the color of the tubing, the less resistance it offers.) You can do a variety of moves with these anywhere.

✓ **Use free weights, or try the weight machines at the gym.** Dumbbells are effective strength training tools. You can do everything from biceps curls (to strengthen the arms) and shoulder lifts (to strengthen the shoulders) to weighted squats (to help boost muscle—and bone—in the legs). Weight machines at the gym are a more advanced way to build bone; book an appointment with a trainer to learn to use them.

To get started, warm up for 5 to 10 minutes to warm up the muscle, helping to prevent injury. Choose a weight or resistance level that will tire your muscles after 12 repetitions. (When you can do more than 15 reps without tiring, increase the amount of weight or resistance.) And plan to do two to three, 20- to 30-minute sessions a week.

(6) It strengthens muscle and bone. Between the ages of forty and eighty, an estimated 30–50 percent of muscle mass is lost[411] (a condition called sarcopenia), resulting in weakness and reduced ability to carry out everyday tasks. This is just one reason why regular and consistent exercise is critical as we get older, because exercise—both cardiovascular and strength training—can help maintain muscle mass.

Strength training or weight-bearing exercise—using weights in the gym, doing body-weight exercises like push-ups, or doing strengthening poses in yoga or Pilates—is also key to building stronger bones. How? Cells called osteoblasts are critical to maintaining your bone structure. When you do weight-bearing exercise, you're stressing your bones (in a good way). Each time you stress your bones, the osteoblasts lay down new bone tissue to strengthen the points where the bone is stressed. Do regular strength training (for different parts of the body), and the osteoblasts continue to reinforce the bone, over and over again.

(7) It reduces stress. The endorphins that are released during aerobic exercise are certainly one reason why exercise can reduce anxiety. But *all* forms of exercise—from gentle yoga, Pilates, and tai chi to tennis, swimming, and walking to running, cycling, and dance—reduce stress, so there's more to the picture than just endorphins.

Many people describe exercise as meditation in motion; while exercising, your mind is able to wander away from the day's worries—which is sometimes all it takes to start the relaxation process! And with rhythmic exercise, like dance or swimming laps or tai chi, this is even truer.

Overall, it's the effect of everything about exercise that helps with stress: it improves sleep (which is so often disrupted during anxious times), boosts self-confidence (which helps with making decisions that work for you—and makes you happier), and can even lower the symptoms of depression.[412]

(8) It keeps your heart healthy. We so often forget that the heart is a muscle, and, like other muscles in the body, you have to move it—or lose it. A stronger heart is a healthier heart.

Exercise also helps the heart in other ways:

• **Exercise promotes weight loss.** Excess weight puts undue strain on the heart, so losing weight is better for the heart.

• **Exercise reduces overall cholesterol**, which has been linked to clogged arteries, and LDL (or "bad") cholesterol levels in the blood, which contribute to heart disease. It also raises HDL (or "good") cholesterol levels in the blood.

• **Regular exercise promotes lowered blood pressure.** High blood pressure puts strain on the heart and can lead to chest pain and a heart attack.

• **Exercise improves the body's ability to use insulin** to control glucose levels in the blood—a risk factor for diabetes, which is also a risk factor for heart disease.

• **Exercise improves the ability of the blood vessels to dilate**, which results in improved oxygen delivery to the body, the muscles, and the heart.[413]

(9) It improves sleep. If you're stressed, chances are you're not sleeping well. Since exercise reduces anxiety and stress, it makes sense that it can also help with getting a better night of zzz's.

But you don't need to be stressed to gain the sleep benefits of exercise. Numerous studies have shown that moderate-intensity exercise—such as a moderate-paced walk—helps people fall asleep more quickly, sleep longer, and have an overall better sleep quality than before exercising.[414]

(10) It helps you live longer. Researchers are constantly studying the benefits of exercise when it comes to health and longevity. And consistently, they've found that it doesn't take a lot of exercise to achieve big health gains.

In one study from the University of Oxford, in the United Kingdom, researchers found that being physically active a few times per week was enough to lower risks of heart disease, stroke, and blood clots.[415] And what's more, more frequent physical activity didn't appear to lower the risks further. This is great news for those of us who don't have time to formally exercise every day of the week!

Healing Water, Healing Movement

For thousands of years, people have sought relief and renewal—physical, emotional, and even spiritual—by immersing themselves in water. There's no doubt about the healing powers of water—why swimming, with its blissful weightlessness, is an exercise that most people can do at any age. It's also incredibly peaceful and meditative if you're in the pool without a lot of noise or other swimmers.

Swimming is excellent exercise (something most people don't realize) because it utilizes arms, legs, and core, which keeps them toned. And, whether you're doing laps, aqua aerobics, aqua jogging (running in the water), or even aqua kickboxing, you're getting your heart rate up—without the impact on joints or muscles (water acts as a cushion for the body's joints, why it's low impact) that land-based exercises like running or jumping can have.

The water also provides up to 42 percent greater resistance than air—making it the perfect weight-training machine. So if you haven't tried water-based exercise yet, give it a go; you may find that—like me—you love it!

Another study found that just moving for two minutes every hour—instead of being sedentary—was associated with longevity and, more specifically, with a 33 percent lower risk of dying overall.[416] This means just getting up from your desk or chair every hour for two minutes (to take a walk around your office, go up and down a set of stairs, or take a quick walk outside and back) was enough to prolong your life.

Sweat: a potent detoxer? One reason why exercise may be so beneficial: sweat is a form of detoxification. The skin is the single largest organ of elimination in the body. By sweating, as through regular exercise (and even use of the sauna[417]), your skin expels toxins and waste through the pores, which are essentially tiny holes in the skin. The skin, though, is not the only organ of detoxification: the kidneys, the liver, the digestive tract, and the lymphatic system all play a critical role in eliminating toxins, too. (The lymphatic system is a network of vessels and organs that run parallel to the cardiovascular system; its job is to maintain immune function and fluid pressure throughout the body as well as draining off waste products.) Even the lungs are an organ of detoxification: every breath brings in fresh oxygen while the lungs filter out pollution, allergens, and more.

In order to effectively detox, though, you need to be sure you're drinking enough water before and after exercise. Drinking water is important any time of the day, because we're composed mainly of water (estimates say women are composed of 60 percent water and men, 66 percent). Without enough water, the body can't rid itself of toxins through the pores through sweat or through the kidneys (which are responsible for flushing waste from the blood). This is why staying hydrated before and after exercise is even more important.

Consider all this detoxification as the body's way of housecleaning!

What toxins are we talking about? We're constantly exposed to toxins on a daily basis: pollution, pesticides, and processed foods, for example. But the body also produces cellular waste that needs to be removed as well. Lactic acid, produced by the muscles during exercise, is one example.

Your cells also produce waste products if your body is fighting a virus or infection or is under a great deal of stress.

Put all these pieces together, and regular, consistent exercise throughout your life will help you live a longer, happier, disease-free life. Add exercise and a Mediterranean diet together, and you've got a longevity combination that is a win-win for your health.

Why Exercise Is Good for Your Skin

Yes, exercise boosts circulation, sending blood—and with it oxygen and key nutrients—to all cells in the body, including the skin cells. This boost in nutrient-rich blood flow gives us a healthy, radiant postworkout glow.

Exercise also helps carry away waste products from skin cells (and all working cells), helping flush them out of the system.

Exercise and aging: Researchers from McMaster University in Ontario found that regular exercise can actually keep the skin young—and may even help reverse skin aging.[418]

Early studies at McMaster found that, in mice, regular exercise (when given access to running wheels) could stave off the early signs of aging. The researchers then followed up in humans.

What they found is fascinating: those volunteers who exercised at least three hours a week (of moderate or vigorous physical activity) had a healthier stratum corneum—the outermost layer of the epidermis—and a thicker dermis layer. The dermis is the second layer of skin, where connective tissue like collagen and elastin—the structural proteins that keep the firm skin and elastic—is found. What's more: the forty-year-old exercisers had skin that was much younger looking when looked at under a microscope, and much closer to that of twenty- and thirty-year-olds.

One theory of the researchers is that exercise causes the release of substances called myokines that trigger healthy changes in cells. Exercisers had almost 50 percent more myokines in their skin than they did at the start of the study.

Yoga as Exercise

Yoga is a supereffective form of exercise because it helps you breathe, relax, and stretch, which feels amazing. In fact, yoga combines both meditation and motion—making it a good exercise option for busy, stressed people (which includes so many of us today, including me!).

I love yoga for all these reasons and often practice it with yoga videos in my home. You don't need to go to a gym or a class to reap yoga's benefits.

Yoga also exercises the body without putting strain on the muscles, making it appropriate for people at any age, even those with illnesses, disabilities, and disease (when other forms of exercise may not be an option).

But the question so often comes up: can yoga *really* provide the health and cardiovascular benefits of exercise like an intense cardio workout can? The answer is yes—but it depends on what kind of yoga you're practicing.

Here's a guide to the different types and the body benefits they provide (keep in mind, though, that many classes—and even yoga videos—can mix different styles into one session):

Ashtanga yoga: This is the most vigorous form of yoga, as it involves doing yoga poses—standing, seated, back bends, and inversions (where a pose has you hold your head below the heart)—one after the other in rapid, flowing movements without much of a break. (It also goes by names like Vinyasa, power, or power yoga.) If you're looking for calorie burn, this is often the best option.

In one study, an hour of beginner Ashtanga yoga was compared with walking on the treadmill for twenty minutes.[419] The study found that Ashtanga yoga was a good cardiovascular workout, revving up heart rate to the level of a moderately brisk walk. Intermediate and advanced classes, researchers theorized, could provide even more vigorous exercise.

Bikram yoga: This is a form of yoga performed in a heated room (typically 105 degrees with 60 percent humidity), which is why it's often called hot yoga. Heat warms the muscles, allowing for greater stretching. This is why Bikram yoga—which often runs through a series of twenty-six postures, each performed twice during a ninety-minute session—has been found to be effective in increasing shoulder, back, and hamstring flexibility.

Hatha yoga: This is one of the most popular forms of yoga and can also go by the names gentle yoga or restorative yoga. This involves slowly moving in and out of poses with controlled breathing. While not necessarily aerobic, hatha yoga does challenge almost every muscle in the body, particularly when you hold your poses for long periods of time. One study found that hatha yoga was better than aerobic exercise at improving balance, flexibility, and strength.[420]

Iyengar yoga: This type of yoga emphasizes physical alignment and makes use of bolsters, straps, blocks, blankets, and other props to help you get into the proper physical position. Iyengar can improve strength, stamina, balance, and flexibility. One study found that people with chronic lower back pain who practiced Iyengar yoga had significantly less disability, pain, and depression after just six months.[421]

Many yoga poses—because they require you to lift your own body weight to balance—strengthen muscles and bones, too. And yoga gets your blood flowing, helping boost circulation.

What's more, a recent study found that regular yoga—no matter what kind you do—can prevent and even reverse the effects of chronic pain on the brain.[422] While other forms of exercise may trigger pain, yoga goes beyond that and actually reverses pain. Pretty amazing! Yoga is an exercise that most people can do for a lifetime.

Making Exercise Fit into Your Busy Life

We all live very busy lives—and it's hard to fit everything we need to do into twenty-four hours in a day. I know this. I experience this every day, juggling my family and my work and my own needs.

But without exercise, all the other parts of the healthy beauty and longevity equation can't work as well. So this is one part you can't skip.

Here are some of the tips that I give to my patients when they need advice about fitting exercise into their schedules:

✓ **Do what you love.** If you hate running, don't tell yourself you have to get to the gym to run on the treadmill. That's a sure reason why you'll skip the gym any chance you get. Find something you love to do—and then go out and do it. Haven't found your fitness love yet? Explore and try new things; you'll find something—even a workout class you never thought you'd love—that's a passion. Once you find that passion, you'll find yourself wanting to exercise, and after doing it, you'll be happier than ever.

✓ **Walk your way healthy.** Sometimes, one of the most enjoyable activities is to lace up your walking shoes and just get outdoors in your neighborhood after dinner, on weekends at the local park, or on a beautiful trail out of town. If you do no other activity, just by walking for at least thirty minutes every day you could rev your heart rate, breathe in fresh air, and clear your mind. According to the American Heart Association, you can reap plenty of health benefits, too, including:[123]

- Reducing the risk of coronary heart disease
- Improving blood pressure and blood-sugar levels
- Improving blood lipid profiles
- Maintaining body weight and lowering the risk of obesity
- Enhancing mental well-being
- Reducing the risk of osteoporosis
- Reducing the risk of breast and colon cancer
- Reducing the risk of non-insulin-dependent (type 2) diabetes

✓ **Mark it on your schedule** as you would a meeting or a big event. We schedule meetings and can't cancel them—exercise is just as important. In fact, I would say it's even more important, because it's critical to your health and your life. Book it, make it nonnegotiable, and you'll have a better chance of doing it.

✓ **Establish goals.** Figure out what you hope to gain from exercise—weight loss, improved health, reduced anxiety—and write it down, so when your motivation is waning, you can look at this and have renewed inspiration.

✓ **Change things up.** Even if you love what you do, if you do it day in and day out, you'll get bored. It happens to even the most motivated among us! Change the course you're running, change the music you're listening to, and most important, change up your workout throughout the week.

✓ **Do just five minutes if that's all the time you have**. You'll feel better having done something—and who knows; you may want to keep going after that!

Our bodies are meant to move, just as they're meant to eat healthy foods. Do your body a favor; get out there and exercise. You definitely won't regret it.

➔**Where do you go from here?** We've talked so much about eating the right foods, destressing, and exercising. It's time to move on to the next step for a healthier, more beautiful you—and that's sleep. It's absolutely critical for your health and your skin. You'll find out just why it's so important for you, and how to get better sleep, in the upcoming chapter.

CHAPTER 4

Get the Sleep You Need

"Sleep is the golden chain that ties health and our bodies together."

~ *Thomas Dekker*

Think about a time when you didn't get enough sleep: either you went to bed way too late, or you just couldn't fall—or stay—asleep. The next day you were tired and groggy and probably reaching for more sugar and caffeine to keep your eyes open and your energy levels up. You were probably too tired to exercise, too. Your skin probably had a dullness to it. You probably didn't feel very beautiful, either. All the healthy habits you've put into place so far are usually the first things out the window after a sleepless night. We've all been there. With two young kids—and having gone through rigorous medical school and training—I've definitely had my share of sleepless nights. And it's very hard to cope with, particularly when I have to be up early at work the next morning!

One or two sleepless nights here and there is to be expected with all that we're juggling today. But what's becoming all too common is the overwhelming insomnia—consistent lack of quality, restful sleep night after night (including enough zzz's overall)—that people are experiencing today. An estimated fifty to seventy million people in the United States today experience what's called a "sleep or wakefulness disorder," according to the Centers for Disease Control and Prevention (CDC).[424]

So what's going on? Why can't people sleep? Researchers spend millions of dollars trying to answer this question and fix the pervasive insomnia in our society. But the main reason people can't get enough sleep has everything to do with our lifestyle.

Think back to the simple Ikarian or Okinawan lifestyles we've talked about throughout this book. These healthy people get plenty of fresh air; nutritious, homegrown food; regular exercise outdoors walking and going about their active daily lives; and daily companionship through friends and family. They also have little persistent stress. They're not "glued" to their smartphones 24/7, checking work e-mails, or even sitting in offices until late in the evening—stressed.

Their simple lives may not work with the rhythms or dictates of a modern work-oriented society, but they work with the natural rhythms of the human body. They nap during the day if they're tired, and when night comes, they eat a light dinner (something that's directly opposed to an American style of eating) and go to bed. And when they go to bed, they sleep easily and soundly with little interruption.[425]

Our work-life patterns are competing with the natural rhythms of our bodies, keeping us awake at night and groggy during the day. And even if you say you function great on just four hours of sleep a night, your body is keeping track when it comes to your health. Long term, you may pay the price in terms of chronic disease and longevity. This is not to scare you; it's to give you the information you need to create the life and the health that you want and your body craves. You need sleep to keep your body, your brain, and your skin healthy.

And if you're taking a pill to help you get to sleep and stay asleep (as almost nine million Americans do[426]), I can tell you that this isn't a good idea. When you understand how the body works—and why allowing your circadian rhythms to get into sync is so important—it's easy to see how our health is tied into all of this. Take a sleeping pill, and you're forcing your body into slumber without fixing the reasons why it can't sleep in the first place. Short term, it seems great: you're sleeping, and you feel energized during the day. But long term, these pills, both prescription and nonprescription, can wreak havoc on your body—and your mind, as studies show.

Researchers found that over-the-counter sleep aids and certain antihistamines used to help sleep increase a person's risk of developing dementia and Alzheimer's disease.[427] Prescription pills—particularly a popular class of antianxiety/sleep medications called benzodiazepines—are no better. These medications are also associated with a higher risk of Alzheimer's disease.[428]

Why Your Body Needs Sleep

There's a reason it's nicknamed "beauty sleep": restful sleep makes a huge difference in the health of the body, as well as in the health and radiance of the skin. Jason* is a patient of mine who is prone to an outbreak of herpes simplex virus around his lips. I know immediately when he comes in with an outbreak that he's been working around the clock and hasn't been sleeping. Then there's Alyson*, another patient of mine: she has eczema—something we're able to keep under control when she's eating right, exercising regularly, and getting enough sleep. As soon as her lifestyle gets hectic (as it often does for this working mom), the eczema flares up. Ditto for my patients with alopecia areata (hair loss), psoriasis, and acne.

The quote at the beginning of this chapter says it all: "Sleep is the golden chain that ties health and our bodies [and skin, I'll add] together."

It keeps us healthy and keeps our mind sharp. In children and teens, it's during sleep that growth and development primarily occurs. It's during sleep that the body does its repair work. It's when the body's energy supplies—depleted during the day—are restored. It's when muscle tissue is rebuilt and restored. It's also when growth hormones are secreted—critical for rebuilding tissue.[429]

As one preeminent sleep expert, Neil B. Kavey, has said:

> *"Think of the body as a car. No car can keep going and going and going without a tune-up or oil change. If it's not tuned, the car may keep running, but not as smoothly as it did when it was maintained properly. You can think of sleep as your body's daily tune-up.*
>
> *"Human beings can function without a full tune-up, but they will be in a state of relative sleep deprivation and won't be able to work or to think as well as they do when they are fully rested. It's like an engine that gets only four out of eight spark plugs replaced and then runs sluggishly."*

Sleep is essential for just about every single process that occurs in the body. Losing just one night of sleep, in fact, has been shown to alter the circadian clock genes in your tissues—which regulate metabolism and even glucose tolerance.[430] More specifically:

Sleep keeps your brain sharp. Sleep is critical for normal functioning of the brain, says research from Oxford University.[431] According to the Oxford sleep scientists, sleep serves as the "brain's housekeeper," helping restore and repair the brain. Poor sleep over time, they found, causes brain shrinkage and problems with reasoning, planning, memory, and problem solving. In fact, one study found that losing just half a night of sleep makes memories less accessible in stressful situations.[432]

This all makes perfect sense. It's during sleep that your brain is forming new pathways to help you learn and absorb new information. (This is why it's often recommended that you rest after you've learned something new—in school or after learning a new skill.) Studies show that sleep helps us focus and remember information (sometimes by the strengthening of neural connections that form our memories).[433]

~ BEYOND BEAUTY TIP ~
Take a Nap!

One thing that the people of Okinawa and Ikaria—and the Mediterranean—know: the benefits of an afternoon nap. This is part of their daily lives—and may be just one reason why they tend to live so long.

It turns out that these island and Mediterranean people are on to something: taking just a short "power" nap during the day, particularly when you're sleepy, has the power to restore you and your health. One study found that a short, 30-minute nap could restore hormones to their normal levels, reducing stress and boosting the immune system. Napping, say researchers, gives the body a chance to recover from the effects of sleeplessness—key to maintaining your health.

How, though, do you fit a nap in to a busy workday? It's not easy, but not impossible either! If you have an office, shut the door (and your eyes) during your lunch hour, but set the timer on your computer or phone so you wake up after 30 minutes. (When I was a resident in the hospital, I used to set a timer so I could nap in the doctor's lounge on my break.) Or, if you don't have an office or a lounge where you can nap, save your catnaps for the weekends (something that I do now).

But *all* aspects of sleep are important for the brain. Research shows that rapid-eye-movement sleep, or REM sleep (a stage of sleep during which dreaming most frequently occurs) plays an important role in learning new information. Deep, restorative sleep is also important, because this is where the brain processes and consolidates newly acquired information.[434]

Enough sleep also helps us make better decisions (our judgment is impaired without enough restful slumber): we're better able to assess a situation, plan accordingly, and choose the correct behavior.[435] Without enough sleep, we're not focused, we're less attentive, and we're less likely to learn and process facts. These are all good reasons to get more zzz's!

Sleep keeps your heart healthy. Lack of sleep is a risk factor for cardiovascular disease along with a poor diet, lack of exercise, and smoking. Researchers have found that not getting enough shut-eye is linked to heart attack and stroke.[436] In fact, these researchers found that nearly 63 percent of their study participants who had a heart attack also had a sleeping disorder. They found that those with sleeping disorders had up to a four-times-higher risk of stroke than those who get enough sleep.

Sleep makes you happier. Not getting enough sleep can affect your mood, making you tenser, more nervous, and more irritable.[437] Chronic insomnia may also increase the risk of developing depression or an anxiety disorder. Having a negative mood can impact relationships at work, at home, and with friends and family, contributing to stress and unhappiness.

In fact, one Swedish study found that not getting enough sleep contributes to higher job-stress levels, a feeling of loss of control at work, and more emotional overreactions on the job.[438] I would venture a guess that these results hold true for everything in our lives outside of work, too. So if you're not sleeping and not loving your job or your life, make solving your sleep issues a priority first.

But the sleep-stress cycle can go round and round: having more tension and anxiety (often from work) can keep you up at night, creating a never-ending cycle of sleep loss (why the stress-busting techniques I mention in chapter 2 are critical). Get enough sleep on a regular basis, and your feelings and mood will stabilize[439]—and your life, overall, will too.

Sleep keeps you at a healthy weight. There have been numerous studies done on the effects of the lack of sleep on weight. One study found that losing just thirty minutes of sleep per night can cause you to gain weight and affect both insulin resistance and your metabolism (slowing it down).[440] Other research found that sleeping less than five hours a night is associated with cravings for more and higher-calorie, carbohydrate-rich foods, triggering weight gain.[441] In fact, research has shown that people eat, on average, about three hundred calories more per day when they're tired.[442] (Anyone who's ever been tired doesn't need research to confirm this!)

But why do you gain weight when you're tired (besides eating more sweets and treats)? Research shows that fatigue-triggered weight gain has everything to do with hormones, which seem to go haywire when you don't get enough shut-eye. Losing just a few hours of sleep a few nights in a row is enough to trigger immediate weight gain.[443] This sleep deprivation increases levels of a hormone called ghrelin, which increases hunger, and lowers levels of a hormone called leptin, which is the hormone that tells you to stop eating because you're full or satiated. What that means: you're less likely to resist the urge to eat unhealthy junk food!

Getting enough sleep also keeps your metabolism—your fat-burning furnace—stoked, which can help you keep obesity at bay. A team of researchers at the University of South Carolina and Arizona State University found that metabolism can be slowed even when you lose just two critical hours of sleep three nights in a row.[444] Add this to your carbohydrate cravings, and you've got a surefire recipe for weight gain.

Sleep helps you live longer. Sleep deprivation (even just one night) has been linked to biological aging.[445] Additional research from the University of California, San Diego, also found that women who got five hours or less of sleep a night didn't live as long as women who got, on average, 6.5 to 7.5 hours of sleep a night.[446] This contradicts the well-known advice to get eight or more hours of sleep a night. Keep in mind that everybody is different. What may work for some ([e.g., five hours a night) won't work for others, like me; I find that I need at least eight hours of sleep a night to function—and be in a happy, energetic mood—the next day.

One study also found that *too* much sleep—particularly for people with weight problems—could be a risk factor for type 2 diabetes.[447] This makes sense. Spend too much time in bed and not enough time moving around, and you could be at risk for even more health problems than just diabetes. The key is moderation—as it is with eating, exercise, work, and just about everything in life—and finding what works best for *your* body.

Sleep helps curb inflammation. Inflammation, as I've mentioned earlier in this book, is linked to everything from heart disease to premature aging. But studies show that lack of sleep—specifically, six or fewer hours a night—triggers high blood levels of inflammatory proteins. One study, in particular, found that one marker of inflammation, called C-reactive protein, is actually higher in people who get six or fewer hours of sleep every night.[448] (This is the protein that's linked to a greater risk of heart problems.) Bottom line: you could eat the healthiest foods and exercise every day, but without enough sleep, you won't be as healthy as you could be. You could also be plagued by skin problems or visibly accelerated signs of aging.

Sleep helps you perform better physically. One fascinating Stanford University study found that college basketball players who slept at least ten hours a night for five to seven weeks ran faster, improved shooting accuracy, and improved overall game performance.[449] But you don't have to be a star basketball player to reap the benefits of sleep. These same study findings can be extrapolated to your everyday physical performance, even if it's just how far you're able to walk in the morning or how you perform in a community 5K.

Sleep reduces stress. Get enough sleep, and whatever is triggering your anxiety just won't seem that insurmountable anymore. Sleeping gives the body a chance to relax and rest without being overwhelmed by worry.

But the opposite is true, too: lack of sleep increases anxiety and stress. In one study, tossing and turning just one night was enough to increase levels of stress hormones like cortisol by the very next evening. Experience sleep loss night after night, and your stress levels—including levels of stress hormones and ACTH, the chemical messenger in the body that tells the adrenal gland to release even more stress hormones—skyrocket.[450]

In fact, some researchers have found that after just one night of sleep deprivation, people had an increase in levels of norepinephrine, a key hormone and neurotransmitter that increases the body's heart rate, blood pressure, and blood sugar in response to stress.[451] Mayo Clinic researchers also found, separately, that prolonged periods of shortened sleep increase a person's blood pressure and heart rate at night, two major risk factors for heart disease.[452]

I've found that just the thought of not sleeping is enough to cause patients to develop enough anxiety to not sleep again the following night. And the cycle repeats itself over and over until patients come in to see me about a particular skin condition that's gotten worse—and I find out they haven't gotten a good night's sleep in weeks or sometimes months! In these cases, I give my patients this mantra to repeat (and believe) to reduce the stress they're feeling. It can help!

"I get plenty of sleep every night, and my body appreciates how I take care of it."

What's more: by getting enough sleep at night, the body is able to take a break from the stress hormones of the day, giving the body a chance to relax and rejuvenate itself. Not getting enough sleep keeps these stress hormones on overdrive—which triggers chronic stress and all the health problems that go along with it.

Sleep increases pain tolerance. It turns out that people who have insomnia or other sleep disturbances also have increased sensitivity to pain. Researchers have found that a reduced tolerance to pain was 52 percent higher in those people who reported having insomnia more than once weekly.[453]

They're not sure why, but these sleep scientists theorize that a neurotransmitter—dopamine, which plays a role in many functions including movement, memory, attention and focus, problem-solving, anxiety, and pain processing—may be affected by the lack of sleep.

Sleep boosts the immune system. Getting adequate amounts of sleep keeps the immune system functioning properly. In one study, researchers found that a lack of sleep caused a reduction in the number of white blood cells called granulocytes, which are critical to immune function.[454] Just one night of sleep deprivation also lowers levels of something called interleukin-6, an antiviral protein.[455] These are two reasons, researchers theorize, that a lack of sleep contributes to illness and chronic diseases like diabetes.

Another study, published in the journal *Sleep*, found that those people who averaged between seven and eight hours of sleep a night were sick less often[456]—something I know I can attest to personally. When I get enough sleep—along with eating healthy, meditating, and exercising—I rarely get sick. But lose a couple of nights of sleep to a busy schedule, and I easily catch the cold that's been passed around my kids' school!

Sleep keeps you safe. Not getting enough sleep, and the drowsiness that occurs as a result, has been found to impair driving performance even more than alcohol.[457] According to the National Highway Traffic Safety Administration, being tired accounted for the highest number of fatal single-car off-the-road crashes.[458] If you're tired, don't get behind the wheel—or pull over when it's safe to do so, so you can take a break.

Sleep improves your skin. Not only do you feel and think better (e.g., more creatively along with having a sharper memory) after getting a restful night of sleep, you also look better. Researchers found that when our circadian clock, which regulates our sleep-wake patterns, among many other things in our body, is out of sync (e.g., from traveling or going to bed and waking at irregular times), skin aging (think fines lines and wrinkles, roughness and dryness, and dull skin) is accelerated, as is our risk of cancer.[459] This is a pretty compelling argument to get enough shut-eye every night.

How to Get a Good Night's Sleep

You know all the reasons why sleep is so critical for the body, but now how do you get to sleep—particularly when you've got so much going on during the day, and in your mind at night? This is a topic I commonly discuss with my patients.

It's one thing to understand *why* sleep is important, but if you still can't get quality shut-eye at night, your health—and the health and appearance of your skin—will suffer. So that's why I put together these sleep-better tips. I know they work, because they're the same ones I give to my patients, and, from what they tell me, they get results. (They work for me, too!)

✓ **Move your body every day.** Study after study shows that physical activity during the day helps you fall asleep more quickly at night, sleep longer, and have overall better sleep quality.[460]

This research comes as no surprise to me; moving your body (which is what we're biologically designed to do) helps tire you out—particularly if you're outdoors in the fresh air. One group of researchers found that 150 minutes of exercise every week (this amounts to about 20 minutes of exercise per day) helps people sleep more soundly at night and feel more alert during the day.[461] Another group of researchers found that certain types of exercise—what they call "purposeful" activity, that is, activity that promotes an end goal—promote sleep better than others, namely walking, biking, yoga, running, weight lifting, and even gardening.[462] This is the type of activity that the Ikarians and Okinawans make a point to do every day.

Be cautious about exercising right before bedtime, unless you're doing gentle, relaxing yoga stretches or rhythmic tai chi. Vigorous aerobic exercise before bedtime boosts circulation and could end up revving you up—and keeping you awake at night.

✓ **Eat a light dinner.** The Ikarians and Okinawans—and even Mediterraneans today—eat their heaviest meals early in the day, saving their lightest meals for evening. Soup, vegetables, and salads with a slice of bread are common meals in the evening—not the large-portioned heavy dinners (often eaten late, after people get out of work) that are so common in America. If you eat too much, your body spends most of its energy digesting food at night, when it should be relaxing—something that can interfere with restful sleep.

✓ **Create a consistent sleep schedule that works for your life.** A set bedtime—when you can realistically go to bed every night, based on your work, your family, and your life—is a must. Consistency is important for proper functioning of your circadian rhythm; it helps your body understand when it's time for sleep.

Your sleep schedule might even include meditation at night to help relax you and your thoughts before bedtime, reading a book, giving yourself a gentle massage, or having a cup of herbal (not caffeinated) tea. Rituals are important, because they help relax the body and mind—and prepare it for sleep.

For this reason, it's also important to have a set wake time every day (even on weekends). Sleeping in or catching up on sleep on weekends throws off your circadian rhythm and may affect how well you sleep as you get back into your workweek.

✓ **Keep your room cool.** Rooms that are too hot or too cold can make you feel uncomfortable and can disturb your sleep. The ideal temperature, say experts, is sixty-five degrees.[463] I personally prefer the room temperature around seventy to seventy-five degrees, but what's important is to find a temperature that's most comfortable for you.

✓ **Shut down electronics at night.** Don't leave your smartphone—or your computer—by your bed. (If you need an alarm clock, use a battery-powered one instead.) And power everything down at least one or two hours before you go to bed. A National Sleep Foundation survey found that kids who leave their electronic devices on at night sleep an hour less than kids who shut off their devices.[464] The same holds true for adults, says other research.[465] The reason has everything to do with the blue light that emanates from these devices, which can interfere with the body's production of the sleep hormone melatonin.

Study after study has found that the blue light that emanates from electronics—your TV, your computer, your smartphone, your e-reader—can affect your circadian rhythms[466] (the internal body clock I mentioned earlier that tells you when to sleep and regulates other critical body processes).

Every one of us has something called photoreceptors in our eyes that register and process light before sending it to the brain. The brain reacts to blue light by suppressing the production of melatonin (because it mimics the wavelengths of natural daylight). This is a hormone secreted by a small gland, the pineal gland, in the brain. Melatonin is released as darkness sets in at night; the more melatonin we have in our system, the sleepier we get. Our body starts to repress the production of melatonin once the sun starts to rise in the morning—so we can wake up and not feel groggy. Melatonin controls sleep and wake cycles and is essential to our circadian rhythms.

Blue light—which is omnipresent in our households and work environments—confuses the brain and our circadian rhythms about whether we should be awake or asleep. The result: persistent sleeplessness and insomnia (which many people try to "fix" by taking sleep medications).

By shutting off your devices before bed, you may find that you fall asleep quicker and stay asleep longer. One University of Colorado study done with campers—out in the wilderness with no exposure to any artificial light (including the blue light emanating from electronics)—found that the campers slept longer and more soundly without exposure to lights than they did when not camping.[467] And we don't need a study to know that the Ikarians and Okinawans don't have or use their smartphones and computers all day long!

The bottom line: health starts with maintaining synchronized circadian rhythms. They're critical to not just sleep: this body clock is essential for our health, our happiness, our well-being, our weight, and even our ability to stave off chronic diseases like diabetes and depression.

✓ **Find ways to relax.** Stress and anxiety are pervasive in our modern society and are key reasons people have trouble sleeping. Meditation, sitting quietly at night and just deep breathing, taking a short nighttime stroll outdoors, and avoiding the news right before bedtime—which is a big source of stress—are all good ways to power down the body and the mind before sleep. Everyone is different, so experiment to see what works best for you, and put it into regular practice.

✓ **Try drinking tart cherry juice.** Cherries are chock-full of health-promoting antioxidants, which are important for the body and for the skin. But one particularly interesting study has now found that the unsweetened juice of tart cherries may help you sleep better, too.[468]

This research shows that drinking eight ounces of juice made from Montmorency tart cherries, twice daily, helps you get eighty-four more minutes of sleep per night. Why? Tart cherry juice contains naturally occurring melatonin—the hormone that helps maintain the body's circadian rhythms and is therefore critical to sleep. (Montmorency cherries have the highest concentration of melatonin of all tart cherries.) I also want to add to make sure you drink organic tart cherry juice, so you can avoid the potential pesticide residue on cherries.

✓ **Be sure you're getting enough vitamin D.** If you're having trouble sleeping, it might be a good idea to have your vitamin D levels checked by your doctor. A deficiency of this vitamin has been linked by numerous researchers to many health-realted problems, including sleep issues.[469] If you're deficient, you can try eating more vitamin D–rich foods like fatty fish (such as salmon), fortified milk or orange juice, or mushrooms (mushrooms produce vitamin D when exposed to light). Or, on the advice of your doctor, you may want to take a vitamin D_3 supplement.

Melatonin and Your Skin

Melatonin—the so-called sleep hormone—also turns out to have beneficial effects on the skin. Have enough of it coursing through your body (one benefit of having a healthy sleep/wake cycle), and you may experience these skin benefits:[470]

Protection from the sun's ultraviolet (UV) light: Melatonin is able to help suppress UV-induced damage to skin cells—thanks to showing off strong antioxidant activity in UV-exposed cells. This doesn't mean that getting enough sleep—or having enough melatonin in your body—eliminates your need for daily sunscreen (more on this in the next chapter). It just means that melatonin offers additional protection for your skin.

A healthier stress response in the skin: We talked about what happens in the skin under stress. Because melatonin is a free-radical scavenger—and a broad-spectrum antioxidant—it seems to help moderate the effect of stress, both external and internal, on the skin. This could, in turn, help reduce the skin problems that develop as a result of stress.

One downside of melatonin, which is why I don't recommend taking supplements: in some people, it seems to activate the skin's pigment-producing cells (called melanocytes), which can darken the skin.

The Five Healthy Stages of Sleep

In ancient times, darkness came, and people went to sleep. They woke with the dawn to start their days. Doing so helped them honor—and align—their internal body clock, which ensured the proper production of the sleep hormone melatonin. Production of the stress hormone cortisol naturally lowers at night, gradually increasing throughout the night to help promote alertness in the morning.[471]

Aligning our body clocks to modern society is hard to do (many people are just getting out of work when it's dark, and others work night shifts), which is wreaking havoc on our sleep patterns and our health.

Getting enough melatonin allows for five healthy stages of sleep; going through all five stages (one full sleep cycle) allows for truly restful, health-promoting sleep. Most people—if getting enough sleep—go through all five of these stages four to six times a night.[472]

These five stages of healthy sleep are:

Stage 1 The lightest stage of sleep—where you feel yourself drifting off. It usually lasts for five to ten minutes. (This is also typically the last stage of sleep before you wake up, if you wake up naturally.)

Stage 2 This stage is when brain activity slows down, as does body temperature. It lasts for about twenty minutes.

Stage 3 This is the start of deep sleep and is typically when blood pressure drops, breathing slows down, and muscles become relaxed. (It's sometimes combined with stage 4 in discussions of sleep.) Stages 3 and 4 can last, together, for about an hour, though it takes up less time as you move through the night.

Create a Bedroom Conducive to Sleep

The ancient Chinese art of feng shui—or arranging your home for better health—has some ideas, below, on how to arrange your sleep space for better slumber.

✓ **Choose the right paint color.** Paints with soft, neutral tones—from soft white and spa blue to warm chocolate brown—help you relax better than vibrant, energetic colors like orange, red, or yellow. And when choosing a paint for the home, opt for low- to no VOC paints; these contain less harmful chemicals called Volatile Organic Compounds (VOC's), which can trigger breathing difficulties, particularly in those prone to asthma.

✓ **De-clutter your space.** Excess stuff, particularly in the bedroom, is often a sign of insecurity and fear—and can contribute to anxiety. According to feng shui principles, clutter in the bedroom—and particularly under the bed—can make you anxious and my just keep you awake at night.

✓ **Don't place mirrors in your bedroom.** Mirrors, according to feng shui, reflect and indicate movement, which can create restless energy—and may inhibit sleep.

✓ **Don't hang chandeliers or ceiling fans above your bed.** According to feng shui, it's a threat to you (something you subconsciously may be aware of and anxious about)—and bad for your health (and sleep)—to have anything hanging over your head as you sleep.

✓ **Ditch the TV in your bedroom.** I've already discussed how using electronics around bedtime can interfere with sleep, but feng shui believes that TVs give off restless energy, even when they're not on, which can trigger insomnia. If you have to have a TV in your bedroom, place it in an armoire or cabinet that you can close off when you go to sleep. (And don't watch it for one to two hours before bed.)

✓ **Have a few plants, but not too many.** One is fine, but too many plants—according to feng shui— symbolize growth and movement, interfering with the peaceful energy you want in the bedroom.

Stage 4 This is the stage where you experience the deepest and most refreshing aspect of sleep—and is when the brain is the most relaxed. It's when the body does its repair work and rejuvenation. It's also when blood supply to the muscles increases and growth hormones are released.

In India's ancient Upanishads—a collection of fundamental spiritual teachings that are central to Hinduism and to self-realization, yoga, and meditation—it's this stage of sleep that offers "a deep state of utter peace wherein Awareness rests unto Awareness, without any egoic sense of body, mind, or world,"[473] where we let go of the body, mind, ego, plans, and concerns and are free in deeply peaceful contentedness.[474]

It's this stage of restorative sleep that some people believe is the most important for body, mind, and spiritual restoration each night.

Stage 5 This is called active sleep or REM (rapid eye movement) sleep—and is when you dream. It's during this stage of sleep (which occurs about ninety minutes after you first fall asleep—and recurs every ninety minutes, getting longer later in the night[475]) that your blood flow, brain activity, and breathing increases, and muscles become fully relaxed and immobilized. (Some experts believe this happens so we can't act out our dreams.)

If any of these stages are cut short—or if the overall number of cycles is reduced—the body doesn't have time to repair and restore itself. Over time, this repeated sleeplessness wreaks havoc on every aspect of our body, including our spirit.

➔**Where do you go from here?** A healthy body and youthful, radiant skin depend so much on your internal state of health and well-being. What you eat, how you manage stress, how you move, and how you sleep are all critical components of your health—and the state of your skin.

Follow the tips and advice that I include in all these previous chapters, and you're on your way toward living a healthy life. But when it comes to healthy beauty, the last component is what you do to your skin physically, from the outside. That's what I'm going to address in the last chapter of this book. Keep reading!

CHAPTER 5

Rejuvenate Your Skin from the Outside

"Glamour is about feeling good in your own skin."

~ *Zoe Saldana*

A healthy body equals radiant, glowing, and healthy skin. This is something that I've talked about throughout this book. It's the reason that I've focused on eating healthy, managing stress, exercising, and getting enough sleep *before* discussing the things that you do to the outside of your skin. I know that when you're healthy and feeling good, you have more confidence in yourself. Your skin is glowing, thanks to all that healthy eating and circulation-boosting exercise. This translates into wanting to take better care of yourself—and your skin.

Without these first healthy Beyond Beauty steps, whatever you do to the outside of your skin won't produce lasting beauty—no matter how much money you spend on pricey facials and exfoliating treatments, injectables, lasers, and skin-care products.

In fact, the goal of skin beauty is not to make your skin "look" younger with temporary makeup and creams but to actually make your skin younger in how it looks and functions. The goal is to restore the physiological function of the skin. A proper skin regimen is age reversing—bringing back radiance, elasticity, firmness, smoothness, and even coloring. Good skin health is just as important as whole-body, mind, or spirit health.

Think about your goals at the beginning of this book. If you've been slowly putting into motion the healthy-living steps I've talked about here, you're probably seeing real changes in your skin already. Maybe the monthly breakouts you've always experienced have become less frequent. Maybe someone you haven't seen in a long time remarked how great you look. Maybe it's all about you: maybe you're embracing your newfound health and energy and feeling more confident and happy in your own skin. Good for you! (You may want to take another selfie at this stage and compare it to your picture when you first started.)

If you haven't had a chance to put into practice the steps I've laid out in the first part of this book, definitely revisit them and circle, highlight, or bookmark whatever healthy habits you're going to take up today. Remember: you don't have to do everything all at once; that would overwhelm even the most motivated person. Instead, pick out small habits to start changing, one at a time. I cannot emphasize enough the importance of these early steps when it comes to radiant, youthful, and beautiful skin.

For many people, these healthy-living steps may be all that they need. Maybe a few tweaks to your daily beauty routine at home, and you're on your way to a lifetime of beautiful skin—no intensive skin rejuvenation necessary. For others, something more—be it more intensive at-home skin-care products or in-office dermatologist procedures—might be the next step to keeping skin at its youthful best. That's what I'll be talking about in this chapter: the steps and healthy habits you can add to your daily routine to help keep your skin looking its youthful best.

Why Do We Age?

As we get older, all the processes in our body start to slow down. This is dictated by our genes—but it's also dictated by the onslaught of our environment and how we live every day in our bodies. I've talked earlier about how free radicals in the environment create a process called oxidation in the body. If you ever cut an apple on a cutting board and left it for an hour, when you return you'll see that the apple has turned brown. That's because of oxidation. That same process occurs inside our bodies (one reason I'm such a big proponent of feeding your body from the inside with a healthy Mediterranean diet full of free-radical-fighting antioxidants).

This oxidation, as well as the normal aging process, shortens telomeres in our body. Remember, these are the plastic tips on the shoelaces of each of our cells that hold our chromosomes together and prevent them from "fraying" at the ends. The longer our telomeres are in our cells, the more youthful they are. The shorter they are, the older our bodies are. These same telomeres exist in each and every one of our skin cells.

Intrinsic and extrinsic aging: There are two types of aging: intrinsic and extrinsic. Intrinsic (which means "from the inside") aging has to do with your genes: the characteristics of aging that you got from your parents, your grandparents, your great-grandparents, and on down the line.

Many patients talk about the genes they inherited from their parents or grandparents. But our genes—and how we age—go back much further in our lineage. Our genes go way back to our historical ancestors. Though it's hard to know how your ancestors aged, a good place to start is seeing how your mom or dad (or grandparents) aged, as this will be a starting point to assess how you'll age, too. Keep in mind, your lifestyle and habits may be much different from those of your parents or grandparents, which may make a difference in how you grow older.

Then there's extrinsic aging (which means "from the outside"); this has everything to do with the environmental factors that surround you. What kind of diet do you eat? How often are you exposed to ultraviolet radiation? How much stress are you under (and how are you managing it on a daily basis)? Do you get enough sleep at night? Do you suffer from chronic illness? Do you smoke, or work or live in an environment with secondhand cigarette smoke? Do you work in an industry with chemical, radiation, or smoke exposure?

Free radicals: the cause of graying hair? Hair gets its color from melanin—the pigment that also determines skin color. There are two types of melanin: eumelanin (dark brown and black) and phaeomelanin (red and yellow). It's the combination of these two types that creates the variety of hair colors—from red to black—that we know today. When hair loses this pigment, it becomes gray, silver, or white. The graying process occurs when there's a buildup of hydrogen peroxide in the hair cell. Hydrogen peroxide is a free radical naturally found in small amounts in hair cells.

The body produces an antioxidant called catalase to keep the hydrogen peroxide in check by converting the hydrogen peroxide to oxygen and water. As we age, however, the body produces less catalase, so the hydrogen peroxide is allowed to build up and block the normal synthesis of hair pigment or melanin.

One compelling study showed that chronic stress—and the long-term production of stress hormones in the body—can damage DNA and cause premature aging and gray hair.[476] There have also been studies showing that smoking (and free-radical production) is linked to premature skin aging and early hair graying. More studies need to be done, however.

Scientists made an interesting discovery when researching vitiligo, a disease where skin loses its pigment and develops white patches. They found that vitiligo occurs from a large amount of oxidative stress on skin-pigment cells from an accumulation of hydrogen peroxide. The same mechanism is responsible for both hair and skin whitening.

The answer to graying hair, I believe, lies in antioxidants, though this is definitely an area in need of further research.

Antioxidants—Why They Make a Difference

As I've mentioned throughout this book, free radicals are highly destructive molecules in our bodies (including in our skin) that can destroy cells and, over time, trigger diseases like cancer. Free radicals are missing an electron, which is necessary to keep them stable. They attack other cells in an effort to steal or donate an electron, pairing up their own odd electron, and in doing so, they trigger a domino effect, creating even more destructive free radicals in the process.

Antioxidants stop free radicals in their tracks by providing the free radical with the extra electron it needs. This stabilizes the free radical, neutralizing it and rendering it harmless. But it's important to note that if you have cancer, some studies have shown that cancer cells are able to turn antioxidants against the body, helping cancer thrive (this is why it's important to talk to your doctor before supplementing with antioxidants).[477]

I cannot emphasize enough how important antioxidants are to our bodies and to our skin. Simply put, antioxidants are nature's great neutralizers. As one group of researchers put it, "a balance between free radicals and antioxidants is necessary for proper physiological [bodily] function."[478]

Our body's antioxidants: With antioxidants being so critical to balance in our body, it makes perfect sense that nature has provided our bodies with their own set of free-radical-fighting antioxidants. These include enzymes with superscientific names like superoxide dismutase, catalase, glutathione peroxidase, and glutathione reductase.

Nonenzymatic antioxidants in the body include alpha lipoic acid, glutathione, vitamin C, vitamin E, and coenzyme Q10 (these are also common supplements today, but the body manufactures its own supply).

All these antioxidants are designed to neutralize free radicals that our body is exposed to. But sometimes—particularly in a modern society with plenty of pollution and pesticides—our bodies' systems can get overwhelmed. When our antioxidant defenses get overwhelmed, it creates a state of oxidative stress in the body. Over time, prolonged oxidative stress can lead to disease.

Other powerful antioxidants: We can supplement our body's stores of antioxidants to shore up our defenses against free radicals, keeping our body—and our skin—healthy. Minerals like selenium, manganese, copper, and zinc, as well as vitamins like A, C, and E, are all antioxidants.

Other antioxidants, which I've talked about throughout this book, include something called phenolics—health-promoting substances found in brightly colored fruits and vegetables, red wine, coffee beans, tea, propolis, and grains. These make up one of the most numerous and widely distributed groups of substances in the plant kingdom, with more than eight thousand phenolic structures known. Not only are phenolics antioxidants, they're also natural anti-inflammatories, antivirals, antibacterials, and anticarcinogenics—pretty powerful plant essences!

– **Another reason to drink green tea.** Green tea is chock-full of health-promoting antioxidants—and there's plenty of research to show that it has numerous health benefits. But green tea also helps the skin: when applied to the skin, it can help calm redness and decrease skin inflammation. When ingested, it also seems to help protect against damage from the sun's ultraviolet (UV) rays.

One study, published in the *British Journal of Nutrition*, found that drinking two cups of green tea every day (along with taking the antioxidant vitamin C) can reduce the effects of UV radiation on the skin.[479] According to researchers, the antioxidants—or catechins—in green tea seem to make the skin more resilient to the effects (including redness) of the UV rays, thereby helping prevent premature aging of the skin and possibly even skin cancer. But this doesn't mean you can drink green tea and forget the sun-precaution tips (including wearing sunscreen every day) that I mentioned earlier. This is just additional protection to keep your skin at its healthy, radiant best.

– **Resveratrol: the antiaging antioxidant?** There may be a reason the Ikarians incorporate red wine into their daily diets. Resveratrol is a potent antioxidant (found in red wine, grape juice, peanuts, and ripe berries) and free-radical scavenger. In plants, it helps protect the plants from damage from the sun's ultraviolet light (which the Ikarians would get a lot of, from being outdoors) and other environmental stressors, as well as helping plants to stave off infections.

What's more, resveratrol—when used topically—has been shown to work synergistically with vitamin E to help stave off the domino effect of skin-cell changes that result from the natural aging process and things like ultraviolet light, pollution, and cigarette smoking.[480]

Just as it does for plants in nature, resveratrol also seems to do for the skin: it protects against the onslaught of free radicals and may just keep skin healthier and more youthful looking for longer.

Topical application of antioxidants: Not only can you ingest antioxidants to shore up the body's defenses, you can also apply them topically.

It's been demonstrated that topical antioxidant use can provide additional protection from oxidative damage, slow skin aging, and improve the appearance of the skin.[481]

I prefer antioxidants with multiple ingredients to target and neutralize the five free radicals found in skin: hydroxyl radicals, peroxyl radicals, peroxynitrite radicals, singlet oxygen radicals, and superoxide anion radicals. One antioxidant ingredient is unable to neutralize all five free radicals alone. By combining ingredients, you're able to target multiple issues at the same time. I describe this to patients as multitasking skin care. Some of my favorite antioxidant ingredients are coffee fruit, green tea, vitamin C, vitamin E, coenzyme Q10, and azelaic acid.

In all the earlier steps in the book, we've dealt with so many of the factors involved with extrinsic aging. In this chapter, we deal with the final component: how you're treating your skin on a daily basis.

Why You Need to Stay out of the Sun

Just fifteen minutes of sun can age you. That's what an Australian study found,[482] which is why I advise all my patients to stay out of the sun—or at least slather up with sun protection whenever they're out in the sun. Study after study shows that it doesn't matter how great your genes are; if you're exposed to the sun, your skin will age faster than normal, and you'll be more at risk of skin cancer.

Other research, published in the journal *Clinical, Cosmetic, and Investigational Dermatology*, found that the sun is responsible for the majority (80 percent) of skin aging. Sun exposure causes hyperpigmentation, reduced skin elasticity, and changes in skin texture—along with fine lines and wrinkles. Plus, the effect of exposure to the sun's ultraviolet rays increases with age: after the age of fifty, people who are exposed to the sun look older than their actual age.[483]

What's more: a tan results from injury to the skin's DNA. The skin darkens in an attempt to prevent further DNA damage. This injury can trigger mutations that can lead to skin cancer, the most frequently diagnosed cancer in the United States, with one in five Americans developing it in their lifetime. In fact, the incidence of melanoma (the most dangerous form of skin cancer) is increasing faster than that of any other cancer.

Tanning beds are particularly bad for your skin, because they emit only UVA rays. In fact, tanning beds emit doses of UVA as much as twelve times that of the sun.

But why exactly does the sun trigger so much damage in the skin? One reason is that the sun's ultraviolet (UV) radiation suppresses the immune system, which is why people with herpes break out in cold sores after exposure to the sun. The other reason is that sun's rays penetrate deep into the skin, triggering damage to the cells and to the skin-firming proteins collagen and elastin.

In fact, exposure to UV radiation reduces our collagen production by 80 percent for forty-eight to seventy-two hours, within twenty-four hours of exposure to the sun!

Here's a quick primer on the sun—and how its rays penetrate the skin:

The sun's ultraviolet or UV rays are divided into UVA rays, UVB rays, and UVC rays. All are invisible to the human eye—and all UV radiation can damage the skin's cellular DNA, triggering genetic mutations (which can cause cancer). For years, it was thought that UVB rays were the most damaging to the skin, but it's only been in recent years that researchers and scientists have discovered that UVA rays—and infrared rays—are even more harmful. Take a look at this helpful chart, below, and you'll see which rays penetrate the different layers of skin—and the damage to the skin that occurs as a result.

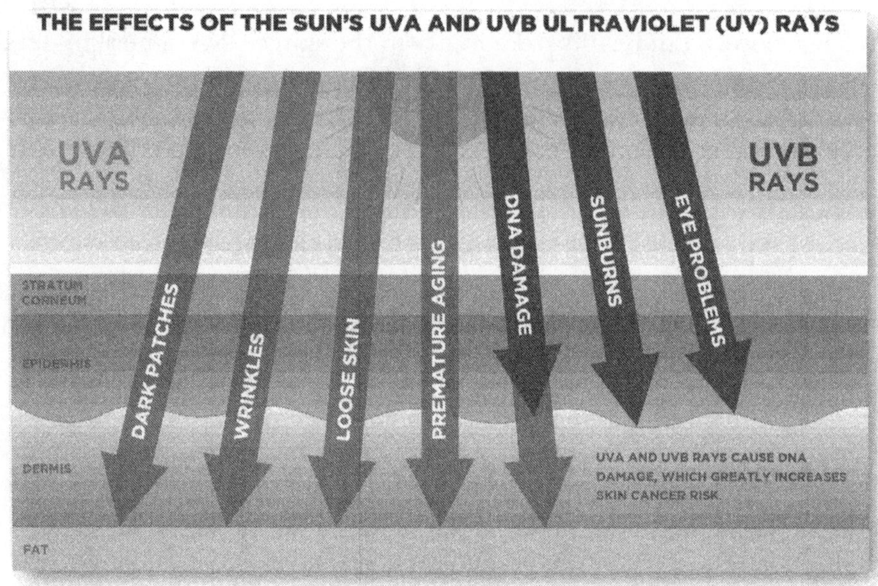

The sun's rays—both UVA and UVB—penetrate deep into the skin's layers, triggering the signs of premature aging as well as skin cancer.

UVA light—or ultraviolet A radiation—is not filtered by the earth's ozone layer, meaning up to 150 percent as much UVA reaches the earth's surface as UVB.

This light penetrates deep into the skin—into the middermis—and is responsible for tanning and also for skin cancer, eye damage (including cataracts), and the breakdown of collagen, the main structural protein responsible for supporting the skin. What's more, these UV rays are present year-round, at all times of the day, and can penetrate through clouds and glass.

A good way to remember what UVA rays do to the skin is that the "A" in UVA is for "aging."

UVB light—or ultraviolet B radiation—is somewhat filtered by the earth's ozone layer, but it only makes up about 4–5 percent of UV light (UVA makes up the rest).

This UV light penetrates less deep than UVA rays; it penetrates to the basal, or bottom, layer of the epidermis, where melanocytes—the cells responsible for pigment—are found. This is the type of light that can cause burning of the skin as well as skin cancer and eye damage (including cataracts). While UVA rays are present at all times of the day, year-round, UVB radiation is most prevalent between 10:00 a.m. and 3:00 p.m., and it doesn't penetrate glass.

A good way to remember what UVB rays do to the skin is that the "B" in UVB is for "burning."

UVC light—or ultraviolet C radiation—is completely filtered out by the ozone layer, so 0 percent of it reaches the earth's surface.

Infrared light: We now have studies showing that infrared (IR) radiation (divided into IR-A, IR-B, and IR-C radiation), thermal heat, and visible light can trigger inflammation and are also responsible for changes in the skin that can lead to premature aging.[484]

New evidence demonstrates that solar aging is a combination of UVA and UVB photoaging (UVA and UVB rays constitute about 7 percent of total solar radiation), visible light aging (almost 40 percent of total solar radiation), infrared aging (about 54 percent of total solar radiation), and thermal or heat aging. Thermal aging occurs from visible light and infrared radiation.

Free radicals are activated by the different parts of solar radiation and heat. The negative effects of solar light on the skin, in the past, were attributed to wavelengths in the UVA and UVB range. But we now know that IR and visible light can also play a part in extrinsic skin aging as well as skin cancer. IR-A radiation, in particular, can penetrate into the skin, reaching the subcutaneous tissues in the deepest layers of the skin. That means it penetrates all the layers of skin, down to fat! IR-B penetrates to the dermis or second layer of skin, and IR-C only enters the outermost layer of the skin, or epidermis.

Infrared radiation also transmits heat energy, which contributes to premature skin aging—as seen on bakers' hands and on the faces of glass blowers.

Visible light, accounting for almost 40 percent of total solar radiation, is able to penetrate to the dermis, generate heat, and produce free radicals.

The problem with infrared light, visible light, and thermal heat is that current broad-spectrum sunscreens don't protect the skin against them. This is why it's so important to layer an antioxidant under the current sunscreens to protect against IR, visible light, and heat—and minimize skin inflammation. Antioxidants have been shown to protect skin cells' DNA, mitochondria, proteins, and membranes—and can help defend the skin from radiation that gets through the sunscreen barrier. Topical antioxidants and sunscreens work together synergistically to protect the skin.

To protect yourself from any of the sun's UV rays:

✓ **Always wear broad-spectrum sunscreen** (this protects against both UVA and UVB rays) whenever you're outdoors, whether it's seven in the morning or three in the afternoon. And do so, too, whether it's sunny or cloudy (the sun's rays can penetrate through clouds).

Ultraviolet rays can also reflect off sand, snow, water, and concrete—so just because you're under an umbrella or covering doesn't mean you don't need sunscreen. And know that if you're in high-altitude areas, there's less atmosphere to absorb the harmful ultraviolet rays, so you're getting more radiation—another reason to apply (and reapply) sunscreen.

✓ **Use enough sunscreen.** You need a golf-ball-size amount of sunscreen (about one ounce or enough to fill a shot glass, though this should be adjusted based on body size) for the entire body every two hours. Most people don't use enough.

✓ **Avoid the sun between 10:00 a.m. and 3:00 p.m.**—when the sun's UVB rays are most prevalent. And seek shade whenever possible.

✓ **Never use a tanning bed.** People who use a tanning bed are 2.5 times more likely to develop a type of skin cancer called squamous cell carcinoma, and 1.5 times more likely to develop a type of skin cancer called basal cell carcinoma. In fact, according to research, when teens use tanning beds, they increase their risk of melanoma (the deadliest kind of skin cancer) by almost 75 percent.[485]

✓ **Consider adding UV-protective film to your car's side and rear windows** (only front windshields typically have it). The sun's UV rays shine through car windows—which is why studies show that the left side of the face in US drivers is more aged in appearance than the right side.[486]

You might also want to add UV-protective film to your house and office windows if you sit near a window all the time (this can help block up to 99.9 percent of UVA radiation).

✓ **Cover up.** Clothing is UV protective. Thicker shirts have more SPF than thinner ones, and darker colors give you more SPF protection than lighter colors. Clothing labeled UPF (ultraviolet protection factor) is also specifically protective against the sun's ultraviolet rays.

✓ **Wear UV-protective sunglasses** whenever you're outdoors to shield your eyes from the sun's damaging UV rays.

I want to make an additional point: with all the information circulating about the benefits of vitamin D, many of my patients are telling me that being out in the sun is actually good for them. Nothing could be further from the truth. While exposure to sunlight does help the body make vitamin D—an essential hormone in the body—I don't recommend getting your vitamin D from the sun because of all the risks from exposure to sunlight. Instead, get vitamin D from your diet or a supplement.

✓ **Live a healthy lifestyle.** It's long been known that exposure to the sun's ultraviolet rays has been linked to the skin cancer melanoma. But now researchers have discovered that lifestyle factors play a role as well. The researchers discovered that something in the skin called microRNAs (or MiRs), which are regulators of genes, become overwhelmed from exposure to things like smoking, air pollution, chronic inflammation, chemicals, a high-fat or high-sugar diet, and a sedentary lifestyle.[487] When these MiRs become overexerted from this exposure, benign melanocytes (pigment cells) can easily transition into melanoma skin cancer. Just another reason why a healthy lifestyle is important to not just a healthy body, but healthy skin, too.

✓ **Get enough probiotics.** I'm a huge advocate of probiotics, as I've mentioned earlier, but there's another reason to take them: more youthful-looking skin. Research shows that probiotics now seem to also protect against photoaging from the sun's ultraviolet B rays.[488] The signs of photoaging include hyperpigmentation, rough skin, fine lines and wrinkles, and sagging skin.

Probiotics seems to work by suppressing water loss from the skin and preventing UVB-triggered changes in the skin like skin thickening and overall skin damage.

You don't necessarily need to take a supplement; you can get probiotics from foods like yogurt and fermented foods like sauerkraut and kefir.

The Visible Signs of Aging

An inverted pyramid (the triangle of youth) is often used to represent a youthful face: healthy, full vibrant cheeks and fullness in the areas around the eyes. As we age, the effects of gravity play a role as everything starts to move downward and we become more of an upright pyramid. We loose the volume in our upper face: from our forehead and cheeks. The eyebrows start to droop and we have excess eyelid folds and wrinkles. Fine lines and wrinkles appear around the mouth, along with a thinning of the lips. There's also a dimpling of the chin. Some of the visible signs of skin aging include:

Dull skin appearance (due to slower skin turnover)

Facial expression lines (how wrinkled you become depends largely on how much sun you have been exposed to in your lifetime)

Telangiectases (small, superficial blood vessels on the surface of the skin)

Dry, rough skin and uneven texture

Laxity or sagging

Irregular brown pigmentation; purpura or bruising

DNA mutations and precancerous and/or cancerous changes in the skin

If you were to look at someone's skin under the microscope (which is what researchers do all the time), certain changes are seen in aging skin, namely:

Thinning of the epidermis, dermis, and subcutaneous fat

Fragmentation & thickening of elastic fibers and collagen

Increased dermal dilated blood vessels

Your Skin: What You Need to Know

Your skin is your finest clothing and the body's largest organ. It covers an average of twenty square feet and weighs about 6 percent of our total weight. Looking at the skin under the microscope, it's made up of three layers (see below). I find that when I explain the skin and its makeup to my patients, they better understand how and why skin aging and skin problems occur—and what they can do to prevent and treat them.

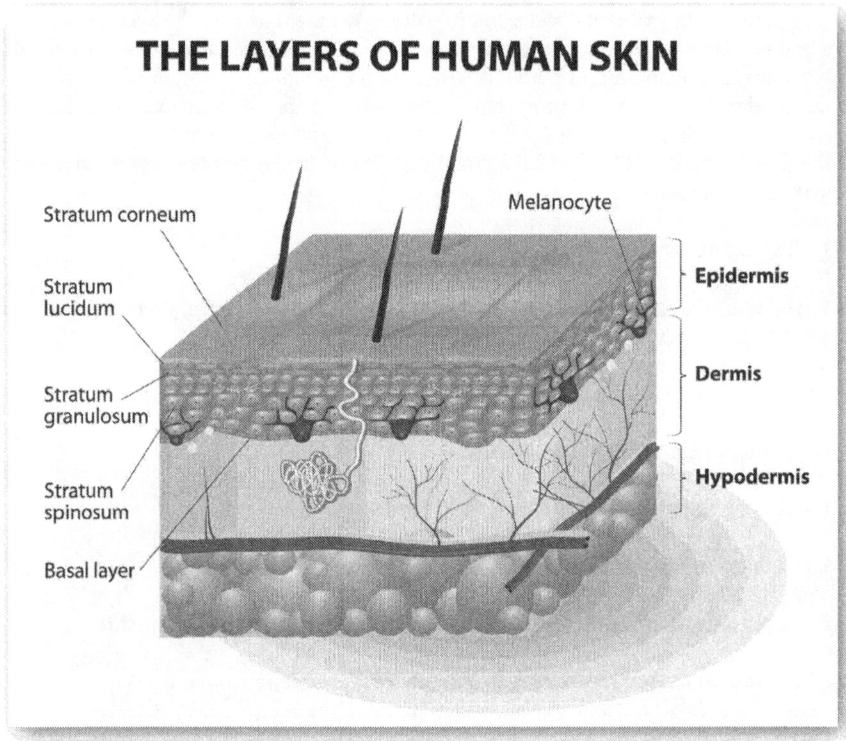

The skin has three layers of skin: the outermost visible layer is the epidermis; the dermis is the second layer; and the hypodermis, containing fat and connective tissue, is the third layer.

The epidermis is the top or outermost layer of the skin. It's extremely thin (only about a tenth of a millimeter in thickness) and is the layer of skin that you see. It helps protect the body from the environment: infections, toxins, and ultraviolet light. (Specialized cells, called Langerhans cells—which are part of the immune system—help protect the skin from infection, but exposure to ultraviolet light can deplete these Langerhans cells.) The epidermis also prevents the skin from water loss.

It's in the epidermis where new skin cells are created. These skin cells are produced in the bottom of the epidermis; they then travel up to the top layer and slough off—creating dead skin cells on the surface of the skin.

It's also in the epidermis that melanin, the pigment that gives your skin and hair color, is produced. Melanin is critical to the skin's protection against the sun's ultraviolet rays. (When the skin tans, it's the body's way of protecting itself.)

The epidermis is thickest on the soles of the feet and thinnest around the eyes and on the eyelids. The outermost layer of the epidermis is called the *stratum corneum.* It's important to keep this layer smooth and exfoliated, as a thickened stratum corneum impairs penetration of skin-care products and gives skin a dull appearance.

The dermis is the second layer of skin that gives the skin its flexibility and strength. It produces sweat, helps you feel (thanks to the nerves present in this layer), grows hair, makes sebum or oil (thanks to sebaceous glands that secrete sebum into hair follicles), and brings blood to the skin through blood vessels.

It's in the dermis that the structural proteins, collagen and elastin, are found. These proteins are what keep the skin youthful looking, firm, and elastic (when you pull on your skin and it snaps back into place, that's a sign of elasticity). It's also in the dermis where hyaluronic acid is found; this helps the skin hold on to water and stay hydrated (this is also what helps our faces retain our youthful fullness).

It's also in the dermis that lymph vessels are found. These transport the lymph fluid that contain white blood cells, which are critical to immune-system functioning.

The dermis is thickest on the back (about thirty times as thick as the dermis on the eyelids).

The subcutaneous layer (or hypodermis) is the bottom layer of skin. It's where fat and connective tissue (which connects the skin to the muscles and the bones) is found, as well as larger blood vessels and nerves—and it's what controls the temperature of the body.

This layer is thickest on the buttocks and abdomen—providing caloric reserves, insulation, and cushioning. It also gives skin its youthful volume. With age, this layer thins and shifts in location.

Your Home Skin-Care Routine

Many first-time patients come into my office interested in fast age-erasing cosmetic procedures like Botox, Juvaderm or other fillers, or even age-erasing lasers, but they do not take care of their skin at home. They don't have a dedicated skin-care regimen or use sunscreen daily.

A simple at-home regimen—cleanse and exfoliate, replenish the skin with key nutrients/ingredients, protect, and moisturize—is the foundation that I recommend for all my patients because it gets results. It's the foundation after putting into practice the healthy-living habits we've discussed in this book, which you can then build on with in-office treatments. It's the foundation that addresses all three layers of the skin: the epidermis, the dermis, and the subcutaneous layer. And it's the foundation that helps repair damage that's already occurred (not to mention, it also prevents future damage).

But keep in mind that while your skin is a reflection of your inner self, it's important to maintain it well all over—not just on the face (which is the area most people are most concerned about). I often advise my patients not to forget the areas that surround the face—the neck, chest, shoulders, and upper back—as well as the lower legs, arms, and hands.

(The skin on the body has a much slower cell-turnover rate than the face, so daily maintenance is needed.) This is why it's important to treat all the areas of the skin with the same maintenance routine and rejuvenation methods. Remember, environmental damage occurs all over the body—though the face is often the most visible.

Here are the key steps that I recommend to all my patients:

Step One

Gently cleanse your skin. Washing your face—morning and night—helps remove makeup and sunscreen, daytime grime that's collected on your face and in your pores, bacteria, dead skin cells, and skin oil. It also preps your skin for any products you're applying afterward, helping them be better absorbed. (Leaving makeup or sunscreen on at night can inhibit the skin's natural exfoliating process, which sloughs off dulling dead skin cells.)

When you're washing your face—or applying any products to the skin—do so gently from the neck upward to the forehead. Applying products in a downward motion tugs down on the skin, which can contribute to sagging over time. Rubbing or tugging at the skin, particularly in the delicate area around the eyes, can also have this effect.

✓ **Be sure to always use a gentle cleanser** (free from chemicals like parabens; propylene glycol; triclosan, an antibacterial; perfumes; and dyes—all of which can irritate sensitive skin). If a cleanser is too harsh, it can strip the skin of natural oils, triggering excess oil production.

You may also need to use a gentle makeup remover before cleansing, particularly around your eyes if you use waterproof makeup. (Not properly removing eye makeup is a sure way to trigger eye irritations.) One of my favorite makeup removers is coconut oil on a cotton ball; it's gentle enough for all skin types—and super effective.

When cleansing around the eyes, gently dab—don't rub—the remover. Since the skin around the eyes is the thinnest anywhere on the body, it's easy to rub and tug and damage this delicate skin, triggering fine lines and deeper wrinkles (called "crow's feet" around the eyes).

✓ **Wash hands before washing your face.** In one study, researchers found that hands contain up to 150 different kinds of bacteria.[489]

✓ **Use lukewarm, not hot or cold, water.** Extreme temperatures strip skin's oils and trigger broken capillaries (blood vessels on skin's surface). Water that's too hot or too cold can also irritate sensitive and rosacea-prone skin.

Why Does pH Matter?

Our skin is designed to protect us—from pollution, from the sun's UV rays, from bacteria and viruses in the environment, and more. But it can only function optimally when the pH of the skin is balanced.

The letters, pH, describe "potential hydrogen" and describes a critical balance between acidity and alkalinity on the skin. If the skin is too acidic (with 1—on a scale of 1 to 14—being the most acidic and 14 being the most alkaline), it's typically red and inflamed or even broken out with acne, rosacea, or eczema. (As we age, our skin becomes slightly more acidic.) If the skin is too alkaline, it's typically very dry and sensitive—and also more prone to wrinkles and sun damage.

The skin should be more acidic (around 5.5 pH), which is optimal for skin health.

The body experiences this same struggle for balance between alkalinity and acidity. Several factors contribute to the acidity or alkalinity of the body—and our skin: the environment around us, our stress levels, the products we put on our skin, and the food we eat (which affects not only the pH levels of the skin, but also the pH levels inside the body). Going back to the Okinawan and Ikarian diets, it's the leafy green veggies, citrus fruits, tomatoes, and beans that offer up the right pH balance inside the body—and on the skin. (Most fruits and vegetables are alkaline in nature. Throw in a cheeseburger with fries and you've just added some acidity into the body.) This is just another reason to eat healthy.

✓ **Gently dab—never rub—skin with a towel to dry.** Harsh rubbing with a towel (or washcloth during the cleansing process) can irritate skin, and over time, the trauma can contribute to fine lines and wrinkles.

✓ **Try a toner.** A toner can help remove any dirt or makeup left behind after cleansing. I'm a big advocate of alcohol-free toners. Alcohol can strip the skin of natural oils, leaving the complexion tight, dry, and in desperate need of moisture. It can also trigger oil production, which—in the case of oily skin, in particular—is not always a good thing.

Keep in mind that a toner is not essential to a skin-care regimen, but I've found that many of my patients like the "clean" feeling a toner can give the skin (some like to use it throughout the day to help reduce shine and freshen skin). Many toners can help restore the natural pH levels of skin.

Look for toners that feed the skin with gentle, natural ingredients like witch hazel, green tea, rosemary, grapeseed, and chamomile. Toners can also contain exfoliating ingredients like glycolic, salicylic, and azelaic acid, which can help slough off dead skin cells, keeping pores clear and the complexion radiant.

Step Two

Exfoliate regularly. The skin is continually renewing itself—shedding dull, old skin cells to make way for newer, more radiant skin cells. This is a process that takes place in the skin every twenty-eight days—though, as we get older, this process slows down. (This is one reason skin looks duller as we get older, particularly if you don't exfoliate regularly.)

The dead skin cells, along with sun exposure, pollution, dirt and grime, makeup, and the skin's oils, all work their way into the skin's pores (tiny holes from which hairs grow), making these pores look larger and potentially clogging them. Exfoliating daily gets rid of this debris on the skin, keeping skin smoother and less likely to break out. Exfoliating has also been shown to help the absorption of the serums, lotions, and creams—particularly those containing the antioxidant vitamin C[490]—that you apply to your skin.

When we exfoliate, the cells in the stratum corneum (that outermost layer of the skin) send signals to the layers of cells below to increase new cell production. This speeds up cell renewal and returns our radiance or youthful glow.

Manual versus chemical exfoliation: There are two ways to exfoliate: manual and chemical. Physical scrubs, electronic cleansing brushes, microdermabrasion, and even cleansing sponges or washcloths are all ways to physically exfoliate the skin. (Microdermabrasion is a technique that exfoliates the superficial layers of the skin with a wand that uses vacuum suction and sand, crystal, or diamond. It takes about thirty minutes and requires little or no healing time.)

A word of caution: scrubs that contain crushed seeds or nut shells are too rough for the face and may cause microscopic tears—along with resulting irritation and inflammation—in your skin.

Chemical exfoliation, on the other hand, sounds unnatural, but it's actually not. There are plenty of natural "chemical" exfoliators in the form of foaming cleansers, home peels, serums, and stronger in-office peels; these work by "ungluing" the gunk from your skin so it can then be washed away.

The most common chemical exfoliators include the following:

- **Alpha hydroxy acids** (AHAs) are acids found naturally in the sugars of plants or milk. There are five AHAs: citric (from citrus fruits), tartaric (from grapes), malic (from apples), glycolic (from sugar cane), and lactic (from milk). They're all water soluble—which means they can't penetrate the skin's sebum (which is why these acids are not ideal for oily skin or skin prone to breakouts). Like other chemical exfoliators, AHAs can increase sensitivity to the sun—another reason to wear SPF daily.

• **Beta hydroxy acids** (BHAs) are essentially salicylic acid, derived from acetylsalicylic acid or aspirin. These differ from alpha hydroxy acids in that they're lipid—or oil—soluble, meaning they're able to penetrate through sebum into pores, exfoliating and getting rid of the debris that can clog pores and contribute to breakouts.

Beta hydroxy acids have been shown to improve the signs of aging, namely fines lines and wrinkles, rough skin, and hyperpigmentation, after at least six months of daily application. But they can also increase sun sensitivity by 50 percent, which means you have to use daily sun protection when you use beta hydroxy acids (but you should be wearing sun protection every day anyway!).[491]

• **Azelaic acid**—which is derived from wheat, barley, and rye—is a jack-of-all-trades, so to speak. It exfoliates the skin, and it's an antibacterial and anti-inflammatory, making it a good option for acne-prone skin. Not to mention it also prevents hyperpigmentation by regulating the production of melanin. Like beta hydroxy acids, it can make skin sun sensitive—so use a daily sunscreen when using products that contain this chemical exfoliant.

• **Retinoids** vary in strength from prescription strength—which go by names like tretinoin (aka Retin-A or Renova) and tazarotene (or Tazorac)—to weaker over-the-counter versions (which go by names like retinyl palmitate, retinol, and retinaldehyde).

I prefer the prescription-strength retinoids, as I believe they're stronger and more effective.

All retinoids are derivatives of vitamin A. These work by sloughing off dead skin cells to prevent pores from clogging, evening out skin tone, and helping prevent premature aging of the skin. They can also stimulate the production of collagen and hyaluronic acid. Retinoids can also make the skin extremely sensitive to the sun (again, why using daily sun protection is an absolute must). These are best used on the skin at night.

When it comes to exfoliating, more is definitely *not* better. Too much exfoliating (e.g., using a manual exfoliator followed by a chemical one, while you're applying retinoids at night) can leave skin irritated. I recommend daily exfoliation to my patients. If this makes skin irritated, then switch to every other day—or every third or fourth day. If your skin can tolerate daily exfoliation, then you can work up to twice-daily exfoliation.

If you're using retinoids on your skin—which can make skin sensitive, particularly if you're using prescription-strength ones—try exfoliating once every three or four days to start. If you can tolerate that, then exfoliate every two days, eventually moving to every day. But if your skin can't tolerate that, then exfoliate every five or six days. The key is to work with your skin; it will tell you what it can tolerate. Then you can adjust your skin-care regimen accordingly.

Step Three

Replenish the skin with antioxidants. I cannot say enough about the benefits of antioxidants—for both the body and the skin.

First, it's important to understand that the skin—like the body—contains its own reserves of natural antioxidants, before you even apply any product with antioxidants. So why then do you need anything else?

The skin's natural antioxidants include vitamin C, found naturally in high levels in both the epidermis and the dermis, where it's critical to the production of the skin-firming proteins collagen and elastin. But these antioxidants are depleted by daily exposure to the sun's ultraviolet rays and to environmental pollution from car exhaust and smoke (including secondhand cigarette smoke).[492] All these things trigger the production of free radicals—unstable molecules, as I've mentioned throughout the book, that can trigger premature aging of the skin and damage to our DNA that can lead to diseases like cancer (including melanoma, one the fastest-spreading and deadliest forms of skin cancer).

What can help: diet and topical antioxidants. One compelling study, in the *American Journal of Clinical Nutrition*, found that eating a diet high in vitamin C–rich foods can actually keep your skin healthier and more youthful looking.[493] Topical antioxidants, on the other hand, replenish the skin's stores from the outside in, thereby helping neutralize the effects of free-radical damage.[494] They also fight inflammation and, in many cases, help the skin stay moisturized. What's more, antioxidants like vitamins C and E have been shown to help prevent UV-induced damage to the skin,[495] keeping the skin youthful looking longer. In doing so, they protect the collagen that you already have and stimulate cells in the skin called fibroblasts (found in the dermis) to produce even more collagen.

Placing antioxidants like vitamin C directly on the skin can offer great benefits by directly targeting the desired areas of improvement. This is why I recommend that all my patients apply topical antioxidants and, when used during the day, layer these antioxidants under a sunscreen.

Some research has shown that pretreating the skin with vitamin C (used *under* a sunscreen) prior to going out in the sun or being exposed to pollution seems to prevent significant free-radical damage (triggered by pollution and the sun's infrared rays).[496]

Why Smoking Ages the Skin

Earlier in this book, I've talked about why smoking (including secondhand and even third-hand smoke) is so bad for your health. No surprise that it's also bad for the skin. Research has shown that the nicotine in tobacco causes blood vessels in our skin to narrow, limiting the oxygen and nutrients it needs and the removal of waste products it doesn't need. The result: delayed wound healing and the production of free radicals that break down the skin-firming proteins—collagen and elastin—as well as DNA. Bottom line: the skin health of smokers is worse than those who don't smoke—and the skin of smokers also ages faster.

The repeated puckering motion of the lips when smoking also contributes to the formation of vertical lines around the mouth.

One study conducted on twins (one who smoked, one who didn't) showed that in the twin who smoked, there was more sagging of the upper eyelids; baggier lower eyelids and bags under the eyes; more facial wrinkles, including between the nose and the mouth (called the nasolabial folds), more wrinkling of the upper and lower lips, and more pronounced sagging of the chin.

I believe e-cigarettes need to be used with caution, too; studies are finding that the vapor from these e-cigarettes still contains chemicals—and with these, you're still puckering up to take a smoke. The best advice I have: find help to quit and then stop smoking for good.

You can find antioxidants in SPF day lotions—but the concentrations of antioxidants in these products aren't as high as I believe they should be to be truly effective. That's why I always recommend that my patients apply a concentrated antioxidant product underneath their sun protection.

When choosing an antioxidant product, look for airless containers that preserve the potency of the antioxidants inside (these containers also keep skin-care products free from bacterial, viral, or fungal contamination). Think about what happens to that apple that's been left out on the counter. The same "rusting" happens to the antioxidants in products, so to speak. Oxygen causes antioxidants to lose their potency. So every time you open your jar or bottle of antioxidants, you're exposing the product to air and decreasing its potency.

Step Four

Apply sunscreen. Sun is the number-one cause of premature aging (which is essentially developing the signs of aging early in life—before your genes dictate it). That's why I recommend that all my patients apply SPF (sun protection factor)—be it in a sunscreen, a foundation, a bronzer, whatever—every single day, rain or shine. And if you're out in the sun, you need to reapply every two hours, or more frequently if you're in and out of the water, sweating, or drying off (which can rub off your protection).

Remember, it's not just the burning UVB rays that you should be worried about. It's the aging and cancer-causing UVA rays—along with infrared (IR) radiation, visible light, and thermal heat—which are present all day, every day, no matter what the weather.

Your SPF should offer broad-spectrum protection; this means it protects against both the sun's aging and cancer-causing UVA rays and burning and cancer-causing UVB rays. Layering an antioxidant under your sunscreen will also help protect against visible light and IR damage.

Sunscreens are divided into two categories: physical and chemical. Each offers protection from the sun but does so in a different way.

Chemical sunscreens work by absorbing ultraviolet radiation. Since they're absorbed into the skin, these sunscreens are more commonly associated with skin irritation. The key to the effectiveness of these products, though, is you need to apply them at least thirty minutes before sun exposure to give them time to work.

One of the most common chemical-sunscreen ingredients is oxybenzone. Something to keep in mind before using this ingredient: Researchers found that this ingredient was actually harmful to the environment, particularly coral reefs (areas where tourism—along with sunscreen use—is high).[497] The study found that oxybenzone triggered DNA damage in adult coral and deformed the DNA in coral in the larval stage, preventing them from developing properly. Coral also suffered bleaching when exposed to the compound.

Physical sunscreens are my favorite; these include titanium dioxide, zinc oxide, and magnesium oxide. They work by reflecting and scattering the sun's ultraviolet radiation. Look for these ingredients in non-nano formulations; these are designed to not be absorbed by the skin (they sit on the skin and act as a physical block) and are well tolerated by people of all skin types—including sensitive skin and rosacea-prone skin. They work immediately upon application, so you don't have to wait before being exposed to the sun.

When looking at a natural sunscreen's label, the ideal concentration of these ingredients is 10–20 percent. The legal maximum is 25 percent, but I often find that these sunscreens are thick and somewhat difficult to wear, particularly on the face.

Step Five

Moisturize as needed. While the skin produces its own oil, called sebum, every skin type still needs to add extra hydration. Frequent skin washing and daily environmental damage can strip the skin of its natural oils.

It's best to apply moisturizer within about three minutes of washing and gently patting dry your skin (this helps prevent any water present in the skin from evaporating). Look for moisturizers that add nutrients, such as antioxidants, back into the skin.

I always recommend that my patients use a moisturizer day and night for optimum hydration. When your skin is properly hydrated, it's even-toned and even-textured, and fine lines and wrinkles are much less noticeable. Nighttime is especially important, as that's when the body undergoes most of its repair—including repair and rejuvenation of the skin. Skin temperature actually rises at night, which can lead to water loss—another reason that moisturizing at night is key. (Rising skin temperature also allows for key ingredients to better penetrate.[498])

Types of moisturizers: There are two forms of moisturizers, humectants and emollients.

Humectants draw water into the outer layer of the skin from the environment and from the deeper dermal layer. These enhance your skin's ability to hold on to water and make your skin feel soft and smooth. One type of humectant is glycerin.

Emollients provide a protective film on skin to prevent water loss; these can be oil or water based. Some types of emollients are natural oils like avocado or safflower oil.

Here's a guide to what moisturizers you should be using for your skin type:

- **Normal/combination skin:** Use a lighter, water-based moisturizer.

- **Oily skin:** Apply a lighter, water-based or noncomedogenic moisturizer (lotions and gels are lighter than creams). Moisturizers with exfoliating ingredients like salicylic or azelaic acid can help keep skin clear.

• **Dry skin:** Use an oil-based cream moisturizer (particularly during cold-weather months).

• **Sensitive skin:** Use soothing ingredients that won't irritate skin; also steer clear of synthetic dyes, synthetic fragrances, and chemicals like phthalates, parabens, and sulfates.

• **Mature skin:** Use an oil-based moisturizer to help add moisture to the skin and hold on to hydration already in the skin.

And whatever you do, don't forget your feet! A common problem I hear about from patients as they age is thickened or callused yellow skin on the feet. The problem is that most people don't care for their feet like they do their face and the rest of their body. But our feet need attention too.

My two-step daily solution: after showering, massage the feet with a pumice stone or other foot scrubber. Then apply a cream or lotion with a chemical exfoliant like glycolic acid (be sure to rub all over your feet, including around your toes). If you can put on a pair of socks afterward to help the cream absorb, do so. The key is to do this two-part regimen every day. You'll see a difference in your feet almost immediately!

Oils: Good for Your Skin—and Your Scalp

Hair is technically dead, but the skin on the scalp is very much alive—and needs regular care. The right oils (look for ones that are 100% pure and organic) massaged into the scalp before washing (cover with a shower cap or towel, and leave on for 30 to 45 minutes) can strengthen the scalp and the hair. Here's a guide:

✓ **Almond oil** is rich in polyunsaturated and mono fatty acids, as well as vitamins A, B, and E. It's an emollient, which means it softens the hair, giving it a silky, lustrous texture. It can also nourish and strengthen the hair—and boost shine.

✓**Argan oil** is extracted from the argan tree (native to the Mediterranean region). It's high in fatty acids and antioxidants like vitamins A and E, which is why it's been used for thousands of years to make hair silkier, softer, and shinier. It's not greasy, which makes it an effective leave-in conditioner.

✓**Avocado oil** is packed with nutrients like vitamins A, B, and E, essential fatty acids, protein, and amino acids (compounds critical to hair growth and strength)—all of which can help feed the hair follicles. Since avocado oil is a humectant (which means it helps lock in moisture), it makes an effective deep conditioner.

✓ **Coconut oil** has been shown to have antibacterial, antifungal, and antiviral properties, thanks to fatty acids called lauric acid and capric acid. It's also rich in antioxidants and nutrients like vitamins E and K. It penetrates deep into the hair shaft, helping to retain moisture, strengthening strands, and keeping hair hydrated.

✓ **Extra-virgin olive oil**—which is chockfull of healthy fats and antioxidants—is an emollient, meaning it gets down deep in the hair shaft, hydrating and adding shine. There's even evidence that using olive oil topically can help prevent hair loss by obstructing production of a hormone, DHT (dihydrotestosterone).

✓ **Jojoba oil**, which comes from the seeds/nuts of the jojoba plant (an evergreen desert shrub), is an emollient wax that's close in composition to human skin oil. It's rich in vitamin E, zinc, and selenium. And it's good for smoothing strands and adding shine.

Your In-Office Antiaging Rx

As I've already mentioned, I always recommend that my patients start first with at-home strategies—changing their diet and their lifestyle, learning techniques to help them destress, starting an exercise program, getting sleep, and tweaking their home skin-care regimen—before having office antiaging procedures done. Sure, I can and do treat patients who are still under stress, don't have time to exercise, and are trying hard to change their love of unhealthy fast food. But these patients won't see lasting changes in their skin and in their radiance if they don't put the other steps into practice first in their life.

I know this personally and have noticed this firsthand with many of my patients. Those who practice a healthy lifestyle—eating a healthy diet, exercising regularly, putting into practice stress-reduction techniques, and regularly using sunscreen—see prolonged benefits from their at-home regimens and in-office procedures. Those who smoke, frequently tan in the sun or in tanning beds, are under mental stress, or eat predominantly junk food are unable to maintain the radiance-boosting and youth-promoting benefits received.

I also recommend repeating this mantra before deciding to have any in-office procedure:

"I love myself exactly as I am. I won't wait to be perfect in order to love myself."

I have found that loving yourself first—and taking care of the body you have—will ensure you are truly happy with yourself, regardless of any in-office technique a dermatologist like me can offer.

The Four-Part In-Office Technique

For aging and skin rejuvenation, I follow a four-part office procedure to target each layer of skin. All these issues must be addressed in order to have more youthful skin.

(1) Target cell turnover. This is where I look at the outermost layer of skin (the epidermis or, more specifically, the stratum corneum) and determine how we can get the dull, dead skin cells to turn over more quickly. This turnover transforms dull skin almost immediately, adding radiance (a result of the more youthful, radiant skin cells underneath showing through). Professional-strength retinoids, peels, microdermabrasion, and lasers are the best ways to achieve more radiant skin.

(2) Even out skin tone. In this part, I'm also targeting the epidermis by addressing hyperpigmentation, increased pore size, and superficial blood vessels (broken capillaries). The best procedures, in office, for this step are professional-strength retinoids and peels, microdermabrasion, and lasers. IPL is also an option; this stands for intense pulsed light. It's not a laser but a light-based treatment that's effective for redness and excess pigment. (The treatment takes around thirty to forty-five minutes and requires one to two weeks to heal. Often multiple treatments are needed, spaced three to four weeks apart.)

(3) Smooth out scarring and wrinkles. In this part, we go deeper into the dermal layer to address scarring and wrinkling with lasers and injectables (like fillers and neurotoxins, such as Botox, Dysport, and Xeomin). The goal is to stop the formation of wrinkles (which neurotoxins do temporarily) and to boost the skin's own production of collagen, which is the skin's scaffolding.

Hyaluronic-acid fillers do this by adding hyaluronic acid back into the skin to fill scars and hollows in the skin. There are many types of fillers, but I prefer hyaluronic acid overall because it stimulates the fibroblasts to produce more collagen at a faster rate. Hyaluronic acid fillers are also used to firm the skin overall, improve fine lines and wrinkles, fill thin lips, add youthful fullness to hollow cheeks, and plump deep wrinkles.

They can also be used to plump the backs of hands, which also lose volume as we age. Most people require one to two treatments per year.

Depending on what needs to be addressed, more aggressive lasers (called fractional lasers) can be performed on the skin.

This is the step where we can also temporarily immobilize certain muscles to prevent wrinkling of the skin; this involves the use of neurotoxins like Botox, Dysport, and Xeomin. To make a muscle contract—be it on the face or anywhere in the body—nerves send signals to the muscles, and the muscles respond by moving. Products like Botox, Dysport, and Xeomin temporarily block the nerve receptors on the targeted muscles to stop only those muscles from moving. This then prevents wrinkle formation in areas like frown lines between the eyebrows and crow's feet around the eyes. The effects last about three to four months.

Can Botox Rejuvenate Aging Skin?

After treating many patients with botulinum toxin A to smooth wrinkles, I've found that the more regularly people do it, the smoother their skin remains. New evidence is now showing exactly why: the advantages of Botox go beyond just smoothing wrinkles.

Long-term benefits: Research is showing that botulinum toxin type A—including Botox, Dysport, and Xeomin (all different brand names for botulinum toxin type A)—not only relaxes muscles and softens fine lines and wrinkles but also seems to rejuvenate aging skin long after it's injected and long after the muscle-immobilizing effects wear off.[499] It seems that this popular injectable also boosts collagen and elastin in the skin, making skin look less wrinkled and younger at the same time.

The lead researcher was quoted as saying: "Studies looking at the ultraviolet damage in the skin have shown minimization of damage with BTX-A, and a link has been established with BTX-A injections and preventing free radical release by the cells—essentially an antioxidant effect. This may account for both the lessening of ultraviolet damage and the improvements seen in collagen and elastin." Further evaluation still needs to be done.

Additional benefits from botulinum toxin type A injections include decreased pain from migraines, decreased sweating, and decreased surgical scars.[500] Other researchers have found that botulinum toxin type A injections improve depression,[501] snoring,[502] and bruxism[503] (teeth grinding).

(4) Address sagging and laxity of skin. In this step, we go into the dermal layer and often into the subcutaneous or fat layer to lift skin. This is why people used to have face lifts years ago, but now we can achieve dramatic results without a lot of downtime. Lasers and fillers (including fat) are now ways to address this aging issue.

Lasers: Lasers, which actually stand for Light Amplification by Stimulated Emission of Radiation, are energy-based treatments that wound the skin and trigger a healing response. They work by directing short, pulsating, concentrated beams of light at the skin. Different lasers penetrate the skin at different levels, depending on the results you want to achieve.

When it comes to the skin, some lasers erase visible blood vessels and redness, while others reduce brown spots, smooth wrinkles, and shrink enlarged pores. Some also target skin laxity by firming the skin, and others can remove hair and even reduce fat. Lasers are pretty amazing jack-of-all-trade tools!

– **Fractional lasers** (one of which is called Fraxel) deliver a series of microscopic, closely spaced laser wounds to the skin. They treat fine lines and wrinkles, enlarged pores, acne scars, and brown spots. The treatment takes about forty-five minutes. As with most lasers, often multiple treatments are needed, spaced three to four weeks apart.

Something worth noting: when antioxidants were applied topically to the skin after a Fraxel laser session, patient downtime (about one week) was reduced by up to two days.[504] It seems that the antioxidants better penetrate into the skin through the microscopic wounds that the Fraxel laser delivers, helping reduce inflammation and redness and heal the skin.

– **Ablative lasers** penetrate deeper and often only need one treatment. They require more healing time, typically seven to ten days, with redness lasting weeks. They also have more risk of loss of pigment and scarring.

Fillers: These work by filling lines, wrinkles, and areas of reduced fat and fullness in the face. There are several categories of fillers—and different brands of fillers within each category. Some fillers are temporary, mimicking the body's own hyaluronic acid, and others are longer lasting. I recommend discussing them with your board-certified dermatologist or plastic surgeon to see which one is right for you. Some of these other wrinkle-smoothing and volume-enhancing fillers include:

Synthetic Fillers

Synthetic fillers are substances created in a lab and are designed to be longer lasting. The downside to these fillers is that if you don't love the look, these fillers can't be reversed as easily as other nonpermanent fillers.

Calcium hydroxyl-apatite: This is a substance naturally found in the bones. When injected into the skin, it can help fill moderate to severe wrinkles and add volume.

• **Radiesse** is a gel filler with calcium hydroxyl-apatite that acts as a scaffolding to help fill and smooth moderate to severe wrinkles and folds on the skin. It can also lift the skin, supplementing the skin's depleted collagen. It can last up to a year.

• **Radiesse (+)** works the same as Radiesse except it contains lidocaine to reduce injection pain. Like Radiesse, it can last up to a year.

Poly-L-lactic acid: This is the same substance that has been used in dissolvable stitches for years.

How to Treat a Sagging Chin?

Laxity of skin on the face can be easily treated with fillers, but loose fat on the chin has been more difficult to address—until now. Something called Kybella® is now being used to correct a sagging chin. Kybella® is an injectable that contains an ingredient called deoxycholic acid that dissolves the excess fat (e.g. a double chin) permanently. (It has to be injected directly into the fat tissue.) Multiple sessions are typically needed to achieve desired results.

• **Sculptra** gradually works over the course of three treatments to smooth shallow to deep wrinkles and folds, with results lasting up to two years. It contains poly-L-lactic acid and works deep in the dermis to help replace lost collagen.

Silicone: This is a permanent filler; it needs to be surgically cut out to remove it. It's controversial because it's been used in non-FDA-approved ways to fill breasts and boost the size of buttocks, with serious side effects. When used by a skilled and experienced physician, though, silicone can be injected—in micro droplets—into wrinkles, helping smooth them and add volume to the skin.

Nonsynthethic Fillers

While many of these substances are created in a lab, all mimic natural substances found in the skin—and can be absorbed into the skin over time with little to no side effects.

Collagen: As I've mentioned, collagen is a critical structural component of your skin. It supports your skin, gives it volume, and keeps it youthful and smooth. But we lose collagen over time, due to aging. Collagen injections replenish the skin's collagen. Collagen comes from human cells and from cows (bovine), though bovine collagen isn't used as much anymore as it requires an allergy test prior to use.

• **Bellafill** (used to be known as Artefill) is typically used to fill the nasolabial folds and severe acne scars on the face. This is actually a non-synthetic filler (it contains 80 percent purified bovine collagen) and a synthetic filler (it contains 20 percent tiny plastic microspheres called polymethylmethacrylate, or PMMA). It also contains pain-reducing lidocaine. The benefit to using Bellafill is it lasts up to five years.

• **Cosmoderm and Cosmoplast** are made from highly purified human collagen. Cosmoderm is used to fill fine lines, wrinkles, and scars that aren't so deep. It can also be used to restore the border of lips. Cosmoplast is used to smooth deeper facial wrinkles and scars. Both are injected into the collagen layer of the skin. Results can last three to six months.

• **Zyderm and Zyplast** are made from highly purified bovine collagen and have been in use since the 1980s. Zyderm is used to smooth fine to moderate lines and wrinkles and shallow scars, as well as restoring the border of thin lips. It can last three to four months. Zyplast is used to smooth more pronounced wrinkles and scars and can last up to a year.

Autologous fat: In these injections, your own fat is removed, via liposuction, from somewhere else on your body and injected into the face to restore volume and smooth facial wrinkles. ("Autologous" means using your own tissues or fat.) The benefit of autologous fat injections is you're not injecting foreign substances into your body. The results can last up to two years or more.

Skin Longevity Filler: Hyaluronic Acid

The skin naturally contains a substance called hyaluronic acid. It binds moisture to the skin, keeping the skin hydrated, plump, supple, and more youthful looking. Technically, it's something called a polysaccharide, which is a carbohydrate. And it's found in the dermal layer of skin. (It's also found in the eyes and in the joints, where it acts as a lubricant.)

But our bodies produce less hyaluronic acid with age—and as we start to produce less, our faces begin to look more gaunt and aged. But fillers like Restylane and Juvéderm—which are the same hyaluronic acid as our body produces, just created synthetically in a lab—can add hyaluronic acid back into the skin, creating the youthful fullness and suppleness that's lost.

One University of Michigan study also found that using these fillers—which last up to a year—can trigger the skin to produce more collagen.[505] The researchers found that the cells in the skin are just happier and more productive when hyaluronic acid is present.

So these fillers are doing more than just superficial filling; it turns out they're helping the skin act in a more youthful manner. The result: younger-looking skin.

There are many different types of hyaluronic-acid fillers. Here's a guide:

• **Belotero Balance** is used to smooth out moderate to severe nasolabial lines (the folds or wrinkles that extend from the inside of the nose to the corner of the mouth).

• **Captique** is used to smooth out moderate to severe facial wrinkles and folds all over the face. It lasts about four months.

• **Elevess** is used to smooth out lines, wrinkles, and furrows all over the face—and was one of the first hyaluronic-acid fillers to contain lidocaine to reduce pain and increase patient comfort.

- **Hylaform** is used to treat moderate facial lines and wrinkles and enhance the lips. It lasts from six to twelve months.

  – **Hylaform Plus** is injected deeper into the dermis than Hylaform, helping smooth out deeper lines, wrinkles, and furrows. It tends to last longer than Hylaform because its hyaluronic-acid particles are larger.

- **Juvéderm:** As of right now, there are five Juvéderm products available:

  – **Juvéderm Ultra and Ultra Plus** are used to smooth out wrinkles and folds, particularly around the nose and mouth. Ultra Plus is a little bit thicker and is typically injected deeper into the dermis—and even the fat layers—to treat more pronounced wrinkles and volume loss. Ultra Plus also tends to last a bit longer (it lasts about twelve months) than Ultra (which lasts nine to twelve months).

  – **Juvéderm Ultra XC and Ultra Plus XC** are used to smooth out wrinkles and folds, particularly along the sides of your nose and mouth. Results last up to one year. These are the same hyaluronic-acid injections as Ultra and Ultra Plus, but they contain the local anesthetic lidocaine to help reduce pain and improve comfort during the treatment.

  – **Juvéderm Volbella XC** is used to increase lip fullness and soften the appearance of lines around the mouth with results lasting up to one year. (This also contains the local anesthetic lidocaine to help improve comfort during the treatment.)

  – **Juvéderm Voluma XC** is an injection that goes deeper into the skin, adding volume to the cheek area. Results last up to two years. (This also contains the local anesthetic lidocaine to help improve comfort during the treatment.)

• **Restylane** is used to add volume and fullness to the skin to smooth out wrinkles (it can also add fullness to the lips) and the nasolabial folds.

Restylane typically lasts four to six months, though depending on the area treated and your own skin, it can last a bit shorter or even longer. As of now, there are four Restylane products available:

– **Restylane L** offers all the benefits of Restylane along with pain-reducing lidocaine for reduced injection pain and increased comfort.

– **Restylane Silk** is specifically designed to plump up thinning lips and smooth the wrinkles and lines around the mouth.

– **Restylane Lyft** (which used to be called Perlane L) treats moderate to severe facial wrinkles, smile lines, and folds in the skin (such as the nasolabial folds). Plus, it can add volume to the cheek area. It contains the local anesthetic lidocaine to help reduce pain and discomfort during and after the treatment. The results last, on average, ten to eighteen months.

• **Perlane** is thicker than Restylane, allowing it to be injected deeper into the dermis, helping treat deeper facial wrinkles and more pronounced volume loss. Because it's thicker, it also tends to last longer than Restylane (about six to nine months).

• **Prevelle** is used for finer lines and wrinkles in more delicate areas of the skin (often making this a good option for first-time users of fillers). It's injected into the upper or middle dermal layer of skin, and lasts three to four months on average.

– **Prevelle Silk** contains pain-reducing lidocaine and is injected deeper into the dermis to smooth deeper lines and wrinkles all over the face, including the nasolabial folds. Prevelle Silk lasts about three to six months.

I want to stress that, even though I offer up all the available in-office options, these are not essential to living a healthy, beautiful, more spiritual, more peaceful, and longer life. What *is* essential is how balanced you are on the inside; how healthy your body, your mind, and your spirit are; and how passionate and invigorated you are by this one beautiful life we have.

➔**Where do you go from here?** Remember that skin is the largest organ in the body. By balancing out what's going on inside the body, you can achieve healthier, more youthful-looking skin.

I know that my clients who put into practice my five-step program in this book look at least ten years younger. And know that it's not about being perfect every day. Sure, we all eat chips or treats once in a while or sleep in and skip our exercise routine. Don't beat yourself up about it. What matters is that you get right back on track and continue the good habits we talk about in this book.

I can't stress enough that the difference you'll feel (more energy, better sleep, more creativity, and more happiness and inner peace) and the difference you'll see firsthand (healthier, younger-looking skin) will be quite dramatic. Even if you never get a single in-office treatment, you'll notice a huge difference by just changing up your lifestyle.

Now, it's time for your final selfie!

Conclusion

Take a look at the lists you put together when you started this book: the healthy habits you wanted to incorporate and the changes you wanted to make. And if you took a selfie, take a look at it. If you haven't made as many changes as you like, remember that inner and outer beauty is a journey, not something that is accomplished just because you finished this book.

This book should serve as a guide: refer back to it regularly as you continue to make changes. As Buddha once said:

"You must make the effort yourself. The masters only point the way."

No one is perfect, not even the Ikarians and the Okinawans! What matters is the progress you make overall and the changes you feel and notice in your own body: how you're sleeping, how you now jump out of bed with energy and enthusiasm in the morning, how you're getting fewer colds, how you're losing weight (without being on a diet), and how your skin glows. By following the tips and advice in this book, you are reinforcing change to your whole person: who you are physically, mentally, emotionally, and even spiritually.

If there's one thing I leave you with, it's that beauty is so much more than just skin deep. It's a reflection of everything we are and everything we do in our lives. When our bodies are truly in a state of healthy balance, it shows on our skin. It also emanates from us in everything that we do: how we relate to others, how much joy and happiness we have in our lives, how much energy we exude, and even how much of our own spirituality we embrace.

Going back to that ayurvedic concept of the ojas, beauty is truly a reflection of the health of our bodies, our minds, our spirits, and our skin.

This is why, as a practicing dermatologist, I advise my patients on lifestyle first before prescribing a medication or administering an in-office treatment. This is also why I look to the Mediterranean lifestyle as a source of proven health- and beauty-promoting secrets. Longevity—the idea that so many of the Ikarian and Okinawan peoples live disease-free for so many years—is inherently tied into beauty…of the body, of the skin, and of the spirit. To recap the steps necessary for true beauty:

✓ **Make over your diet.** Changing up what you eat to resemble a Mediterranean diet will do wonders for your skin. It will help clear up skin problems, help reduce the development of new fine lines and wrinkles (and even help soften the ones you already have), and give you a healthy radiance so often equated with youth.

✓ **Make over your life.** Take a look at what's really important to your health: reducing stress and embracing happiness, exercising, and getting enough sleep. Follow the Mediterranean lifestyle steps I've put forth here to help revamp your life. The difference it will make in your health is dramatic—and the change you'll see in your skin, for the better, will be dramatic as well.

✓ **Make over your skin routine.** Consistency at home is key—as are antioxidants. Put together a regular morning and evening skin ritual that utilizes antioxidants, and you'll notice a difference within days.

Please know that I do not equate beauty with how we look with lots of makeup. Beauty is how we look and feel about ourselves when we look in the mirror in the morning, without makeup. It's about the glow we have in our eyes, the radiance that shines from our skin, and the smile we have in our soul.

Beauty is also the natural confidence we have about who we are without all the external trappings. And beauty is the pureness of our spirit and the joy we gain from our everyday lives with friends and family.

May you enjoy true beauty every single day of your life—and may this book help you along your journey.

** All patient names have been changed to protect their privacy.*

Acknowledgments

I WOULD LIKE TO THANK my husband for his incredible patience and support while I worked on this book—and for believing in me from the start. I would also like to express my gratitude to all my family and friends for their longtime help and guidance as I pursued the career of my dreams.

And where would I be without my patients? You give me joy in my job—and help me to look forward to coming to work every day. You inspire me with your wisdom and your motivation to be your best. Thank you for sharing your stories and allowing me to help guide you. My greatest wish is that this book helps you on your journey to a healthier, happier you.

Thank you, too, Lauren, Debra, Marjorie, Liz, Sabrina, Rachel and Maria for making the office run so smoothly—so I could focus on my patients, my family, and this book. And, Jennifer, Chris, Sam, Josh, Christian, and Jeff, all I can say is I couldn't have picked a better group of teammates!

And to everyone in Lily Dale, New York: Joseph Shiel, John White, Bridghid Murphy, and Joseph Tittel. I can always count on your wisdom to give me new insights to incorporate in my own life—and include in this book.

I would also like to recognize the many teachings and teachers that have influenced my life and my writing: Dr. Andrew Weil, Dr. Wayner Dyer, Dr. Deepak Chopra, and Dr. Mehmet Oz. There's also Caroline Myss, Eckhart Tolle, Michael Singer, and Henry David Thoreau.

And in a greater sense, I am inspired—and continue to be inspired—by the teachings of Jesus, Buddha (Siddhartha Gautama), Mahatma Gandhi, Jalal ad-Din Muhammad Rumi or Rumi, Lao Tzu in the Tao Te Ching, and Krishna in the Bhagavad Gita.

And lastly, thank you to my coauthor, Valerie Latona, for your tireless dedication and endless hours to helping me put my ideas into print. I couldn't have done this without you.

Introduction

1. Ditte Neess, Signe Bek, Maria Bloksgaard, Ann-Britt Marcher, Nils J. Færgeman, and Susanne Mandrup, "Delayed Hepatic Adaptation to Weaning in ACBP–/– Mice Is Caused by Disruption of the Epidermal Barrier," *Cell Reports* (2013), doi: 10.1016/j.celrep.2013.11.010.

Chapter 1: Give Your Diet a Mediterranean Makeover

2. Justin McCurry, "Centenarians Set to Hit Record High of 54,397," *Japan Times*, September 13, 2013, http://www.japantimes.co.jp/news/2013/09/13/national/centenarians-set-to-hit-record-high-of-54397/#.VAWQpcWSyCk.

3. Z. Zadak, R. Hyspler, A. Ticha, et al., "Polyunsaturated Fatty Acids, Phytosterols and Cholesterol Metabolism in the Mediterranean Diet," *Acta Medica* (Hradec Kralove) 49, no. 1 (2006): 23–6.

4. Matti Marklund, Karen Leander, Max Vikström, et al., "Polyunsaturated Fat Intake Estimated by Circulating Biomarkers and Risk of Cardiovascular Disease and All-Cause Mortality in a Population-Based Cohort of 60-Year-Old Men and Women," *Circulation*, June 17, 2015, http://circ.ahajournals.org/content/early/2015/06/17/CIRCULATIONAHA.115.015607.abstract.

5. "Mediterranean Diet Linked with Lower Risk of Heart Disease Among Young U.S. Workers," Harvard School of Public Health, News, February 4, 2014, http://www.hsph.harvard.edu/news/press-releases/mediterranean-diet-linked-with-lower-heart-disease-risk/.

6. Maria I. Maraki and Labros S. Sidossis, "Update on Lifestyle Determinants of Postprandial Triacylglycerolemia with Emphasis

on the Mediterranean Lifestyle," *American Journal of Physiology—Endocrinology and Metabolism*, July 7, 2015, http://ajpendo.physiology.org/content/ajpendo/early/2015/07/07/ajpendo.00245.2015.full.pdf.

7. H. Schroeder, J. Marrugat, J. Vila, et al., "Adherence to the Traditional Mediterranean Diet Is Inversely Associated with Body Mass Index and Obesity in a Spanish Population," *Journal of Nutrition* 134 (2004): 3355–61.

8. "Ogimi Okinawans Sleep Well, Eat Well, and Work Hard," *Centenarian Secrets and Longevity Science*, June 4, 2008, http://centenariansecrets.blogspot.com/2008/06/httpwww.html.

9. Dan Buettner, "The Island Where People Forget to Die," *New York Times*, October 24, 2012, http://www.nytimes.com/2012/10/28/magazine/the-island-where-people-forget-to-die.html?pagewanted=all&_r=0.

10. Demosthenes B. Panagiotakos, Christina Chrysohoou, Gerasimos Siasos, et al., "Sociodemographic and Lifestyle Statistics of Oldest Old People (>80 Years) Living in Ikaria Island: The Ikaria Study," *Cardiology Research and Practice*, February 24, 2011, http://www.ncbi.nlm.nih.gov/pmc/articles/PMC3051199/.

11. Martha Clare Morris, Christy C. Tangney, Yamin Wang, et al., "MIND Diet Associated with Reduced Incidence of Alzheimer's Disease," *Alzheimer's & Dementia*, February 11, 2015, http://www.alzheimersanddementia.com/article/S1552-5260(15)00017-5/abstract.

12. Valerie C. Crooks, James Lubben, Diana B. Petitti, et al., "Social Network, Cognitive Function, and Dementia Incidence among Elderly Women," *American Journal of Public Health* 98, no. 7

(July 2008): 1221–1227, http://ajph.aphapublications.org/doi/abs/10.2105/AJPH.2007.115923.

13. Kristina Orth Gomer, Annika Rosengren, and Lars Wilhelmsen, "Lack of Social Support and Incidence of Coronary Heart Disease in Middle-Aged Swedish Men," *Psychosomatic Medicine* 55 (1993): 37–43, http://wellness.unl.edu/wellness_documents/lack_of_social_support_and_effects_of_coronary_heart_disease.pdf.

14. "Fiber: Start Roughing It!," *The Nutrition Source*, Harvard School of Public Health, http://www.hsph.harvard.edu/nutritionsource/fiber-full-story/.

15. "Fiber Intake Tied to Reduced Kidney Stone Risk," *MPR*, December 30, 2014, http://www.empr.com/fiber-intake-tied-to-reduced-kidney-stone-risk/article/390315/?DCMP=EMC-MPR_DailyDose_rd&cpn=flecmpr, steld, xolderm&hmSubId=&hmEmail=LUGbza6izzVZv4gxnvu2QsU5jYgc1zdl0&dl=0&spMailingID=10276342&spUserID=MzA3NTI4MTQwMjAS1&spJobID=442464700&spReportId=NDQyNDY0NzAwS0.

16. Yang Yang, Long-Gang Zhao, Qi-Jun Wu, et al., "Association between Dietary Fiber and Lower Risk of All-Cause Mortality: A Meta-Analysis of Cohort Studies," *American Journal of Epidemiology*, first published online December 31, 2014, http://aje.oxfordjournals.org/content/181/2/83.

17. F. Sofi, F. Cesari, R. Abbate, et al., "Adherence to Mediterranean Diet and Health Status: Meta-Analysis," *British Medical Journal* 337 (2008): a1344–50, http://www.ncbi.nlm.nih.gov/pubmed/18786971.

18. F. B. Hu and W. C. Willett, "Optimal Diets for Prevention of Coronary Heart Disease," *Journal of the American Medical Association* 288 (2002): 2569–78.

19. "Mediterranean Diet Cuts Heart Disease Risk by Nearly Half," *EurekAlert!*, American College of Cardiology, March 4, 2015, http://www.eurekalert.org/pub_releases/2015-03/acoc-mdc030315.php.

20. "Mediterranean Diet: Good for the Brain Too?," *MPR*, October 23, 2015, http://www.empr.com/medical-news/mediterranean-diet-good-for-the-brain-too/article/448919/?DCMP=EMC-MPR_DailyDose_cp&cpn=flecmpr%2csteld%2cxolderm&hmSubId=&hmEmail=LUGbza6izzVZv4gxnvu2QsU5jYgc1zdl0&NID=1700857323&dl=0&spMailingID=12766652&spUserID=MTgwMTYxMDE2MjI0S0&spJobID=641616286&spReportId=NjQxNjE2Mjg2S0.

21. Nikolaos Scarmeas and Connie Diekman, scheduled presentation, American Academy of Neurology annual meeting, Toronto, April 10–17, 2010.

22. N. Scarmeas, J. Luchsinger, N. Schupf, et al., "Physical Activity, Diet and Risk of Alzheimer Disease," *Journal of the American Medical Association* 302, no. 6 (2009): 627–637.

23. M. De Lorgeril, P. Salen, J. L. Martin, et al., "Mediterranean Dietary Pattern in a Randomized Trial: Prolonged Survival and Possible Reduced Cancer Rate," *Archives of Internal Medicine* 158 (1998): 1181–7, http://www.researchgate.net/publication/13659917_Mediterranean_dietary_pattern_in_a_randomized_trial_prolonged_survival_and_possible_reduced_cancer_rate.

24. G. Buckland, A. Agudo, and L. Luján, "Adherence to a Mediterranean Diet and Risk of Gastric Adenocarcinoma within the European Prospective Investigation into Cancer and Nutrition (EPIC) Cohort Study," *American Journal of Clinical Nutrition* 91, no. 2 (2010): 3810–90, http://www.ncbi.nlm.nih.gov/pubmed/20007304.

25. V. Cottet, M. Touvier, A. Fournier, et al., "Postmenopausal Breast Cancer Risk and Dietary Patterns in the E3N-EPIC Prospective Cohort Study," *American Journal of Epidemiology* 170, no. 10 (2009): 1257–67, http://www.ncbi.nlm.nih.gov/pubmed/19828509.

26. M. Filomeno, C. Bosetti, E. Bodoli, et al., "Mediterranean Diet and Risk of Endometrial Cancer: A Pooled Analysis of Three Italian Case-Control Studies," *British Journal of Cancer* 112 (2015): 1816–1821, http://www.nature.com/bjc/journal/v112/n11/full/bjc2015153a.html.

28. "SPF on Your Plate: Researcher Connects the Mediterranean Diet with Skin Cancer Prevention," ScienceDaily, American Friends of Tel Aviv University, August 17, 2010, www.sciencedaily.com/releases/2010/08/100816122206.htm.

29. I. Shai, D. Schwarzfuchs, Y. Henkin, et al., "Weight Loss with a Low-Carbohydrate, Mediterranean, or Low-Fat Diet," *New England Journal of Medicine* 359, no. 3 (2008): 229–41.

30. I. Abete, D. Parra, and A. B. Crujeiras, "Specific Insulin Sensitivity and Leptin Responses to a Nutritional Treatment of Obesity via a Combination of Energy Restriction and Fatty Fish Intake," *Journal of Human Nutrition and Dietetics* 21, no. 6 (2008): 591–600, http://www.researchgate.net/publication/23226269_Specific_insulin_sensitivity_and_leptin_responses_to_a_nutritional_treatment_of_obesity_via_a_combination_of_energy_restriction_and_fatty_fish_intake.

31. W. C. Willett, "The Mediterranean Diet: Science and Practice," *Public Health Nutrition* 9, no. 1A (2006): 105–10, http://www.ncbi.nlm.nih.gov/pubmed/16512956.

32. M. A. Martínez-González, C. Fuente-Arrillaga, J. M. Nunez-Cordoba, et al., "Adherence to a Mediterranean Diet Is Associated with a Reduced Risk of Diabetes: Prospective Cohort Study," *British Journal of Medicine* 336, no. 7657 (2008): 1348–1351, http://www.ncbi.nlm.nih.gov/pmc/articles/PMC2427084/.

33. A. Sanchez-Villegas, M. Delgado-Rodriguez, A. Alonso, et al., "Association of the Mediterranean Dietary Pattern with the Incidence of Depression: The Seguimiento Universidad de Navarra/University of Navarra Follow-up (SUN) Cohort," *Archives General Psychiatry* 66, no. 10 (2009): 1090–1098, http://archpsyc.jamanetwork.com/article.aspx?articleid=210386.

34. A. Sanchez-Villegas, P. Henriquez, M. Bes-Rastrollo, et al., "Mediterranean Diet and Depression," *Journal of Public Health Nutrition* 9, no. 8A (2006): 1104–9.

35. Minesh Khatri, Yeseon P. Moon, Nikolaos Scarmeas, et al., "The Association between a Mediterranean-Style Diet and Kidney Function in the Northern Manhattan Study Cohort," *CJASN Clinical Journal of the American Society of Nephrology*, October 2014, http://cjasn.asnjournals.org/content/early/2014/10/29/CJN.01080114.

36. X. Gao, H. Chen, T. T. Fung, et al., "Prospective Study of Dietary Pattern and Risk of Parkinson's Disease," *American Journal of Clinical Nutrition* 86 (2007): 1486–94.

37. G. McKellar, A. McEntegart, R. Hampson, et al., "A Pilot Study of a Mediterranean-type Diet Intervention in Female Patients with Rheumatoid Arthritis Living in Areas of Social Deprivation in Glasgow," *Annals of Rheumatic Diseases* 66 (2007): 1239–43.

38. Gabriele Nagel, Gudrun Weinmayr, Andrea Kleiner, et al., "The ISAAC Phase Two Study Group," Institute of Epidemiology, Ulm University, Helmholtzstr, April 6, 2010.

39. R. Barros, A. Moreira, J. Fonseca, et al., "Adherence to the Mediterranean Diet and Fresh Fruit Intake are Associated with Improved Asthma Control," *Allergy* 63, no. 7 (2008): 917–23.

40. Raphaelle Varraso, Stephanie E. Chiuve, Teresa T. Fung, et al., "Alternate Healthy Eating Index 2010 and Risk of Chronic Obstructive Pulmonary Disease among US Women and Men: Prospective Study," *BMJ* 350 (2015), published online before print, http://www.bmj.com/cgi/doi/10.1136/bmj.h286.

41. Elaine Chong, Centre for Eye Research Australia (CERA is affiliated with the University of Melbourne and the Royal Victorian Eye and Ear Hospital, where it is based).

42. C. B. Huang and J. L. Ebersole, "A Novel Bioactivity of Omega-3 Polyunsaturated Fatty Acids and Their Ester Derivatives," *Molecular Oral Microbiology* 25, no. 1 (2010): 75–80.

43. Leo Galland, "Diet and Inflammation", *Nutrition in Clinical Practice* 25, no. 6 (2010): 634–40, http://ncp.sagepub.com/content/25/6/634.full.pdf+html.

44. D. Giugliano, A. Ceriello, and K. Esposito, "The Effect of Diet on Inflammation: Emphasis on the Metabolic Syndrome," *Journal of the American College of Cardiology* 48, no. 4 (2006): 677–85, http://www.ncbi.nlm.nih.gov/pubmed/16904534?dopt=Citation.

45. J. H. O'Keefe, N. M. Gheewala, and J. O. O'Keefe, "Dietary Strategies for Improving Post-Prandial Glucose, Lipids,

Inflammation, and Cardiovascular Health," *Journal of the American College of Cardiology* 51, no. 3 (2008): 249–55, http://www.ncbi.nlm.nih.gov/pubmed/18206731.

46. Diana Ernst, "Certain Food Combos Prevent Weight Gain, While Others Promote It," *MPR*, April 9, 2015, http://www.empr.com/news/certain-food-combos-prevent-weight-gain-while-others-promote-it/article/408263/.

47. "Worried About Prostate Cancer? Tomato-Broccoli Combo Shown to Be Effective," *ACES College News*, College of Agricultural, Consumer, and Environmental Sciences, January 16, 2007, http://news.aces.illinois.edu/news/worried-about-prostate-cancer-tomato-broccoli-combo-shown-be-effective.

48. Rui Hai Liu, "Health Benefits of Fruit and Vegetables Are From Additive and Synergistic Combinations of Phytochemicals," *American Journal of Clinical Nutrition* 78, no. 3 (2003): 517S–520S, http://ajcn.nutrition.org/content/78/3/517S.full.

49. Adam Baer, "The Most Powerful Food Combinations," *Men's Health*, http://www.menshealth.com/mhlists/healthy-food-combinations/Apples_Chocolate.php.

50. G. Shoba, D. Joy, T. Joseph, et al., "Influence of Piperine on the Pharmacokinetics of Curcumin in Animals and Human Volunteers," *Planta Medica* 64, no. 4 (1998): 353–6, http://www.ncbi.nlm.nih.gov/pubmed/9619120.

51. Sally Wadyka, "Inflammation: Skin Enemy Number One," *YouBeauty.com*, September 29, 2011, http://www.youbeauty.com/skin/inflammation.

52. Jonathan I. Silverberg and Philip Greenland, "Eczema and Cardiovascular Risk Factors in 2 US Adult Population Studies," *Journal of Allergy and Clinical Immunology*, published online January 8, 2015, http://www.jacionline.org/article/S0091-6749(14)01677-7/abstract.

53. Emil A. Tanghetti, "The Role of Inflammation in the Pathology of Acne," *Journal of Clinical and Aesthetic Dermatology* 6, no. 9 (2013): 27–35, http://www.ncbi.nlm.nih.gov/pmc/articles/PMC3780801/.

54. Whitney P. Bowe, Nayan Patel, and Alan C. Logan, "Acne Vulgaris: The Role of Oxidative Stress and the Potential Therapeutic Value of Local and Systemic Antioxidants," *Journal of Drugs in Dermatology*11, no. 6 (2012): 742–746, http://www.biomedsearch.com/nih/Acne-vulgaris-role-oxidative-stress/22648222.html.

55. D. J. Betteridge, "What Is Oxidative Stress?," *Metabolism* 49, 2 Supplement 1 (2000): 3–8, http://www.ncbi.nlm.nih.gov/pubmed/10693912.

56. Cristiana Miglio, Emma Chiavaro, Attilio Visconti, et al., "Effects of Different Cooking Methods on Nutritional and Physicochemical Characteristics of Selected Vegetables," *Journal of Agricultural and Food Chemistry* 56, no. 1 (2008): 139–147, http://pubs.acs.org/doi/abs/10.1021/jf072304b.

57. Sharon Barbour, "Cancer Boost from Whole Carrots," *BBC News*, June 16, 2009, http://news.bbc.co.uk/2/hi/health/8101403.stm.

58. Veronica Dewanto, Xianzhong Wu, Kafui K. Adom, and Rui Hai Liu, "Thermal Processing Enhances the Nutritional Value of Tomatoes by Increasing Total Antioxidant Activity," *Journal of Agricultural and Food Chemistry* 50, no. 10

(2002): 3010–3014, http://pubs.acs.org/doi/abs/10.1021/jf0115589; http://www.news.cornell.edu/stories/2002/04/cooking-tomatoes-boosts-disease-fighting-power.

59. M.J. Ceko, K. Hummitzsch, N. Hatzirodos, et al., "X-Ray Fluorescence Imaging and Other Analyses Identify Selenium and GPX1 as Important in Female Reproductive Function," *Metallomics* 7 (2015): 71–82, http://pubs.rsc.org/en/Content/ArticleLanding/2015/MT/C4MT00228H#!divAbstract; "Women's Fertility Linked to Detox Element in Diet," *ScienceDaily*, November 17, 2014, http://www.sciencedaily.com/releases/2014/11/141117111008.htm?utm_source=feedburner&utm_medium=email&utm_campaign=Feed%3A+sciencedaily%2Ftop_news%2Ftop_health+%28ScienceDaily%3A+Top+Health+News%29.

60. Jung Eun Kim, Susannah L. Gordon, Mario G. Ferruzzi, et al., "Effects of Egg Consumption on Carotenoid Absorption from Co-Consumed, Raw Vegetables," *American Journal of Clinical Nutrition*101, no. 1 (2015): 75–83, http://ajcn.nutrition.org/content/102/1/75.

61. Whitney P. Bowe, "Diet and Acne," *JAAD* 63, no. 1(2010): 124–141, http://www.jaad.org/article/S0190-9622(09)00967-0/references.

62. Reena Rupani, "Probiotics for Healthy Skin," *Dermatology Times*, June 4, 2015, http://dermatologytimes.modernmedicine.com/dermatology-times/news/probiotics-healthy-skin.

63. Rodrigo Barros, "The Role of the Skin Microbiome in Health and Disease," *MD Magazine*, February 22, 2015, http://www.hcplive.com/conference-coverage/aaaai-2015/The-Role-of-the-Skin-Microbiome-in-Health-and-Disease?e5=Email_md5&utm_source=Informz&utm_

medium=HCPLive&utm_campaign=Trending%20News%20 2/22/15.

64. Ibid.

65. Vanessa Leone, Sean M. Gibbons, Kristina Martinez, et al., "Effects of Diurnal Variation of Gut Microbes and High-Fat Feeding on Host Circadian Clock Function and Metabolism," *Cell Host & Microbe* 17, no. 5 (2015): 681–689, http://www.cell.com/cell-host-microbe/abstract/S1931-3128(15)00123-7?_returnURL=http%3A%2F%2Flinkinghub.elsevier.com%2Fretrieve%2Fpii%2FS1931312815001237%3Fshowall%3Dtrue.

66. David McNamee, "Metabolic Syndrome May Be Prevented by Healthy Gut Bacteria," *Medical News Today*, November 24, 2014, http://www.medicalnewstoday.com/articles/285962.php; Benoit Chassaing, Ruth E. Ley, and Andrew T. Getwirtz, "Intestinal Epithelial Cell Toll-like Receptor 5 Regulates the Intestinal Microbiota to Prevent Low-Grade Inflammation and Metabolic Syndrome in Mice," *Gastroenterology* 147, no. 6 (2014): 1363, http://www.pubfacts.com/detail/25172014/Intestinal-Epithelial-cell-Toll-like-Receptor-5-Regulates-the-Intestinal-Microbiota-to-Prevent-Low-g.

67. "Microbes Help Produce Serotonin in Gut," *ScienceDaily*, April 9, 2015, http://www.sciencedaily.com/releases/2015/04/150409143045.htm?utm_source=feedburner.

68. **A. Mardinoglu, S. Shoaie, M. Bergentall, et al., "The Gut Microbiota Modulates Host Amino Acid and Glutathione Metabolism in Mice,"** *Molecular Systems Biology* **11, no. 10 (2015): 834,** http://msb.embopress.org/content/11/10/834.

69. "5 Claims About Probiotics and Good Gut Health," *Houston Methodist*, July 22, 2013, http://www.newswise.com/articles/5-claims-about-probiotics-and-good-gut-health.

70. Eamonn M. Quigley, "Gut Bacteria in Health and Disease," *Gastroenterology & Hepatology* 9, no. 9 (2013): 560–569, http://www.ncbi.nlm.nih.gov/pmc/articles/PMC3983973/.

71. Melissa Healy, "When Obesity Is an Inherited Trait, Maybe Gut Bacteria Is the Link," *LA Times*, November 6, 2014, http://www.latimes.com/science/sciencenow/la-sci-sn-obesity-genes-gut-bacteria-20141106-story.html; Julia K. Goodrich, Jillian L. Waters, Angela C. Poole, et al., "Human Genetics Shape the Gut Microbiome," *Cell* 159, no. 4 (2014): 789–799, http://www.cell.com/cell/abstract/S0092-8674(14)01241-0.

72. Jennifer Ackerman, "How Bacteria in Our Bodies Protect Our Health," *Scientific American* 306, no. 6, http://www.scientificamerican.com/article/ultimate-social-network-bacteria-protects-health/.

73. "Diversifying Your Diet May Make Your Gut Healthier," *ScienceDaily*, July 14, 2015, http://www.sciencedaily.com/releases/2015/07/150714142231.htm?utm_source=feedburner&utm_medium=email&utm_campaign=Feed%3A+sciencedaily%2Ftop_news%2Ftop_health+%28ScienceDaily%3A+Top+Health+News%29.

74. Jeff Minerd, "AACR: A Diet High in Cabbage May Help Prevent Breast Cancer," *MedPage Today*, October 31, 2005, http://www.medpagetoday.com/HematologyOncology/BreastCancer/2035; "Sauerkraut, Uncooked, May Prevent Cancer," *Well Being Journal*, https://www.wellbeingjournal.com/sauerkraut-uncooked-prevents-cancer/; H. Szaefer, B. Licznerska, V. Krajka-Kuzniak, et

al., "Modulation of CYP1A1, CYP1A2 and CYP1B1 Expression by Cabbage Juices and Indoles in Human Breast Cell Lines," *Nutrition and Cancer* 64, no. 6 (2012): 879–88, http://www.ncbi.nlm.nih.gov/pubmed/22716309.

75. Kate Johnson, "Probiotic 'Promising' to Prevent and Treat Atopic Dermatitis," *Medscape Multispecialty Medical News*, November 9, 2014, http://www.medscape.com/viewarticle/834650.

76. Rodrigo Barros, "The Role of the Skin Microbiome in Health and Disease," *MD Magazine*, February 22, 2015, http://www.hcplive.com/conferences/aaaai-2015/The-Role-of-the-Skin-Microbiome-in-Health-and-Disease?e5=Email_md5&utm_source=Informz&utm_medium=HCPLive&utm_campaign=Trending%20News%20 2/22/15.

77. Bob L. Smith, "Organic Foods vs. Supermarket Foods: Element Levels," *Journal of Applied Nutrition* 45, no. 1 (1993), http://www.ask-force.org/web/Organic/Smith-Organic-1993.pdf; http://www.organicconsumers.org/Organic/organicstudy.cfm.

78. "Fruit & Vegetable Peel Perks," University of California Berkeley Wellness, http://www.berkeleywellness.com/healthy-eating/nutrition/slideshow/fruit-vegetable-peel-perks.

79. "Environmental Working Group's Shopper's Guide to Pesticides in Produce," http://www.ewg.org/foodnews/list.php.

80. Michael deCourcy Hinds, "Assessing the Effects of Chemically Treated Food," *New York Times*, March 31, 1982, http://www.nytimes.com/1982/03/31/garden/assessing-the-effects-of-chemically-treated-food.html.

81. “Mercury: Health Effects,” US Environmental Protection Agency, http://www.epa.gov/mercury/effects.htm.

82. Jason R. Richardson, Michele M. Taylor, Stuart L. Shalat, et al., “Developmental Pesticide Exposure Reproduces Features of Attention Deficit Hyperactivity Disorder,” *FASEB Journal*, January 28, 2015, published online before print, http://www.fasebj.org/content/early/2015/01/30/fj.14-260901.

83. Crystal Smith-Spangler, Margaret L. Brandeau, Grace E. Hunter, et al., “Are Organic Foods Safer or Healthier Than Conventional Alternatives?: A Systematic Review,” *Annals of Internal Medicine* 157, no. 5 (2012): 348–366, http://annals.org/article.aspx?articleid=1355685&resultClick=3.

84. Sepideh Arbabi Bidgoli, Tara Eftekhari, and Reza Sadeghipour, “Role of Xenoestrogens and Endogenous Sources of Estrogens on the Occurrence of Premenopausal Breast Cancer in Iran,” *Asian Pacific Journal of Cancer Prevention* 12, no. 9 (2011): 2425–30, http://www.researchgate.net/publication/221797477_Role_of_xenoestrogens_and_endogenous_sources_of_estrogens_on_the_occurrence_of_premenopausal_breast_cancer_in_Iran.

85. Diane M. Barrett, “Maximizing the Nutritional Value of Fruits & Vegetables,” University of California, Davis, http://ucce.ucdavis.edu/files/datastore/234-780.pdf.

86. S. Pandrangi and L. F. Laborde, “Retention of Folate, Carotenoids, and Other Quality Characteristics in Commercially Packaged Fresh Spinach,” *Journal of Food Science* 69, no. 9 (2004): 702–707, http://extension.psu.edu/food/safety/publications/laborde-folate.pdf.

87. Graham Bonwick and Catherine S. Birch, "Antioxidants in Fresh and Frozen Fruit and Vegetables: Impact Study of Varying Storage Conditions," University of Chester, http://bfff.co.uk/wp-content/uploads/2013/09/Leatherhead-Chester-Antioxidant-Reports-2013.pdf.

88. "Freezing Blueberries Improves Antioxidant Availability," *Newswise,* July 22, 2014, http://www.newswise.com/articles/freezing-blueberries-improves-antioxidant-availability.

89. Solmaz Barazesh, "Probing Question: How Do Antioxidants Work?," *Penn State News,* August 18, 2008, http://news.psu.edu/story/141171/2008/08/18/research/probing-question-how-do-antioxidants-work.

90. Lien Ai Pham-Huy, Hua He, and Chuong Pham-Huy, "Free Radicals, Antioxidants in Disease and Health," *International Journal of Biomedical Science* 4, no. 2 (2008): 89–96, http://www.ncbi.nlm.nih.gov/pmc/articles/PMC3614697/.

91. V. Lobo, A. Patil, A. Phatak, et al., "Free Radicals, Antioxidants, and Functional Foods: Impact on Human Health," *Pharmacognosy Review* 4, no. 8 (2010): 118–126, http://www.ncbi.nlm.nih.gov/pmc/articles/PMC3249911/.

92. Lien Ai Pham-Huy, Hua He, and Chuong Pham-Huy, "Free Radicals, Antioxidants in Disease and Health," *International Journal of Biomedical Science* 4, no. 2 (2008): 89–96, http://www.ncbi.nlm.nih.gov/pmc/articles/PMC3614697/.

93. Ibid.

94. S. H. Ley, Q. Sun, W. C. Willett, et al., "Associations between Red Meat Intake and Biomarkers of Inflammation and Glucose Metabolism in Women," *American Journal of Clinical Nutrition* 99, no. 2 (2014): 352–60, http://www.ncbi.nlm.nih.gov/pubmed/24284436.

95. Y. A. Cho, J. Kim, A. Shin, et al., "Dietary Patterns and Breast Cancer Risk in Korean Women," *Nutrition and Cancer* 62, no. 8 (2010): 1161–9, http://www.ncbi.nlm.nih.gov/pubmed/?term=Nutrition+and+Cancer%2C+Cho+YA%2C+Korean+women+vegetables%2C+fish.

96. "Red Meat May Raise Young Women's Breast Cancer Risk," Harvard School of Public Health News, http://www.hsph.harvard.edu/news/hsph-in-the-news/red-meat-may-raise-breast-cancer-risk/.

97. Tanushree Banerjee, Deidra C. Crews, Donald E. Wesson, et al., "High Dietary Acid Load Predicts ESRD among Adults with CKD," *JASN*, published online before print, January 12, 2015, http://jasn.asnjournals.org/content/early/2015/02/11/ASN.2014040332.

98. J. W. van Heijst, H. W. Niessen, K. Hoekman, et al., "Advanced Glycation End Products in Human Cancer Tissues: Detection of Nepsilon-(carboxymethyl)lysine and Argpyrimidine," *Annals of the NY Academy of Sciences* 1043 (2005): 725–33, http://www.ncbi.nlm.nih.gov/pubmed/16037299#; K. A. Moy, L. Jiao, N. D. Freedman, et al., "Soluble Receptor for Advanced Glycation End Products and Risk of Liver Cancer," *Hepatology* 57, no. 6 (2013): 2338–45, http://www.ncbi.nlm.nih.gov/pubmed/23325627.

99. "Eating Grilled Meat Increases Risk of Alzheimer's and Diabetes," *Medical News Today*, February 25, 2014, http://www.medicalnewstoday.com/articles/273155.php.

100. K. Puangsombat and J. S. Smith, "Inhibition of Heterocyclic Amine Formation in Beef Patties by Ethanolic Extracts of Rosemary," *Journal of Food Science* 75, no. 2 (2010): T40–7, http://www.ncbi.nlm.nih.gov/pubmed/20492265.

101. "Brush On the Marinade, Hold Off the Cancerous Compounds," *ScienceDaily*, June 28, 2007, http://www.sciencedaily.com/releases/2007/06/070627124111.htm.

102. A. Keys, A. Menotti, M. J. Karvonen, et al., "The Diet and 15-Year Death Rate in the Seven Countries Study," *American Journal of Epidemiology* 124, no. 6 (1986): 903–15.

103. R. W. Owen, W. Mier, A. Giacosa, et al., "Phenolic Compounds and Squalene in Olive Oils: the Concentration and Antioxidant Potential of Total Phenols, Simple Phenols, Secoiridoids, Lignans and Squalene," *Food and Chemical Toxicology* 38, no. 8 (2000): 647–659, http://www.ncbi.nlm.nih.gov/pubmed/10908812.

104. M. I. Covas, "Olive Oil and the Cardiovascular System", *Pharmacology Research* 55, no. 3 (2007): 175–86, http://www.ncbi.nlm.nih.gov/pubmed/17321749.

105. Mahtab Najmi, Zahra Vahdat Shariapanahi, Mohammad Tolouei, et al., "Effect of Oral Olive Oil on Healing of 10–20% Total Body Surface Area Burn Wounds in Hospitalized Patients," *Burns*, published online, October 8, 2014, http://www.burnsjournal.com/article/S0305-4179%2814%2900279-4/abstract?rss=yes.

106. S. Y. Kong, M. Takeuchi, H. Hyogo, et al., "The Association between Glyceraldehyde-Derived Advanced Glycation End-Products and Colorectal Cancer Risk," *Cancer Epidemiolog, Biomarkers &*

Prevention 24, no. 12 (2015): 1855–63, http://www.ncbi.nlm.nih.gov/pubmed/26404963.

107. Ken Branson, "Olive Oil Kills Cancer in Minutes," Health, Futurity.Com, February 19, 2015, http://www.futurity.org/olive-oil-cancer-859862/; O. LeGendre, P. A. S. Breslin, D. A. Foster, "(-)-Oleocanthal Rapidly and Selectively Induces Cancer Cell Death Via Lysosomal Membrane Permeabilization (LMP)," *Molecular & Cellular Oncology*, posted online January 23, 2015, http://www.tandfonline.com/doi/abs/10.1080/23723556.2015.1006077#.VOdArfnF-n9.

108. "Adverse Health Effects of Plastics," Ecology Center, http://ecologycenter.org/factsheets/adverse-health-effects-of-plastics/.

109. S. Jobling, T. Reynolds, R. White, et al., "A Variety of Environmentally Persistent Chemicals, including Some Phthalate Plasticizers, Are Weakly Estrogenic," *Environmental Health Perspectives* 103, no. 6 (1995): 582–587, http://www.ncbi.nlm.nih.gov/pmc/articles/PMC1519124/.

110. "Baby Teethers May Leach Chemicals from Plastics, Study Suggests," *MPR*, May 19, 2015, http://www.empr.com/news/baby-teethers-may-leach-chemicals-from-plastics-study-suggests/article/415466/?DCMP=EMC-MPR_DailyDose_cp&CPN=flecmpr, steld, xolderm&hmSubId=&hmEmail=LUGbza6izzVZv4gxnvu2QsU5jYgc1zdl0&dl=0&spMailingID=11428288&spUserID=MTgxMDI1NzYzMjY4S0&spJobID=541285157&spReportId=NTQxMjg1MTU3S0.

111. John D. Meeker and Kelly K. Ferguson, "Urinary Phthalate Metabolites Are Associated with Decreased Serum Testosterone in Men, Women, and Children from NHANES 2011–2012," *Journal of*

Clinical Endocrinology & Metabolism, August 14, 2014, http://press.endocrine.org/doi/abs/10.1210/jc.2014-2555.

112. Natalia M. Grindler, Jennifer E. Allsworth, George A. Macones, et al., "Persistent Organic Pollutants and Early Menopause in U.S. Women," *PLOS One*, January 28, 2015, http://journals.plos.org/plosone/article?id=10.1371/journal.pone.0116057.

113. S. H. Swan, S. Sathyanarayana, E. S. Barrett, et al., "First Trimester Phthalate Exposure and Anogenital Distance in Newborns," *Human Reproduction*, first published online February 18, 2015, http://humrep.oxfordjournals.org/content/early/2015/02/03/humrep.deu363.abstract.

114. "Bisphenol A (BPA)," National Institutes of Health, National Institute of Environmental Health Sciences, http://www.niehs.nih.gov/health/topics/agents/sya-bpa/.

115. A. Veiga-Lopez, S. Pennathur, K. Kannan, et al., "Impact of Gestational Bisphenol A on Oxidative Stress and Free Fatty Acids: Human Association and Interspecies Animal Testing Studies," *Endocrinology*, January 20, 2015, epub ahead of print, http://www.ncbi.nlm.nih.gov/pubmed/25603046.

116. *Arunoday Bhan, Imran Hussain, Kairul I. Ansari, et al.*, "Bisphenol-A and Diethylstilbestrol Exposure Induces the Expression of Breast Cancer Associated Long Noncoding RNA HOTAIR *In Vitro* and *In Vivo," Journal of Steroid Biochemistry and Molecular Biology, no. 141 (2014): 160–170,* http://www.sciencedirect.com/science/article/pii/S0960076014000314; Pheruza Tarapore, Jun Ying, Bin Ouyang, et al., "Exposure to Bisphenol A Correlates with Early-Onset Prostate Cancer and Promotes Centrosome Amplification and Anchorage-Independent Growth In Vitro,"

PLOS One, March 3, 2014, http://www.plosone.org/article/info%3Adoi%2F10.1371%2Fjournal.pone.0090332.

117. T. Peter Stein, Margaret D. Schluter, Robert A. Steer, et al., "Bisphenol A Exposure in Children With Autism Spectrum Disorders," *Autism Research*, published online January 15, 2015, http://onlinelibrary.wiley.com/doi/10.1002/aur.1444/abstract;jsessionid=73BDF42F83A518D0EC8AEA43E0068D37.f01t01?systemMessage=Wiley+Online+Library+will+be+disrupted+on+7th+March+from+10%3A00-13%3A00+GMT+%2805%3A00-08%3A00+EST%29+for+essential+maintenance.++Apologies+for+the+inconvenience.

118. Sanghyuk Bae and Yun-Chui Hong, "Exposure to Bisphenol A from Drinking Canned Beverage Increases Blood Pressure: Randomized Crossover Trial," *Hypertension*, published online before print, December 8, 2014, http://hyper.ahajournals.org/content/early/2014/12/08/HYPERTENSIONAHA.114.04261.abstract.

119. Johanna R. Rochester and Ashley L. Bolden, "Bisphenol S and F: A Systematic Review and Comparison of the Hormonal Activity of Bisphenol A Substitutes," *Environmental Health Perspectives*, March 16, 2015, http://ehp.niehs.nih.gov/1408989/.

120. Ying-Ying Fan, Jian-Lun Zheng, Jing-Hua Ren, et al., "Effects of Storage Temperature and Duration on Release of Antimony and Bisphenol A from Polyethylene Terephthalate Drinking Water Bottles of China," *Environmental Pollution*, September 2014: 113–120, http://www.sciencedirect.com/science/article/pii/S0269749114002000.

121. "What Should I Limit Sodium," Answers by Heart, The American Heart Association, http://www.heart.org/idc/groups/heart-public/@wcm/@hcm/documents/downloadable/ucm_300625.pdf.

122. "NHLBI Study Finds DASH Diet and Reduced Sodium Lowers Blood Pressure for All," National Heart, Lung, and Blood Institute, December 17, 2001, http://www.nhlbi.nih.gov/news/press-releases/2001/nhlbi-study-finds-dash-diet-and-reduced-sodium-lowers-blood-pressure-for-all.

123. "Elevated Brain Aluminium and Early Onset Alzheimer's Disease in an Individual Occupationally Exposed to Aluminium," *Journal of Medical Case Reports*, February 10, 2014, http://www.jmedicalcasereports.com/content/8/1/41/abstract.

124. Heather B. Patisaul and Wendy Jefferson, "The Pros and Cons of Phytoestrogens," *Frontiers in Neuroendrocrinology* 31, no. 4 (2010): 400–419, http://www.ncbi.nlm.nih.gov/pmc/articles/PMC3074428/.

125. J. H. Mitchell, P. T. Gardner, D. B. McPhail, et al., "Antioxidant Efficacy of Phytoestrogens in Chemical and Biological Model Systems," *Archives of Biochemistry and Biophysics* 360, no. 1 (1998): 142–8, http://www.ncbi.nlm.nih.gov/pubmed/982643.

126. Judy A. Carman, Howard R. Vlieger, Larry J. Ver Steeg, et al., "A Long-Term Toxicology Study on Pigs Fed a Combined Genetically Modified (GM) Soy and GM Maize Diet," *Journal of Organic Systems* 8, no. 1 (2013): 38–54, http://www.organic-systems.org/journal/81/8106.pdf.

127. John Douillard, *The 3-Season Diet: Eat the Way Nature Intended* (Harmony, 2001).

128. G. Parker, N. A. Gibson, H. Brotchie, "Omega-3 Fatty Acids and Mood Disorders," *American Journal of Psychiatry* 163, no. 6 (2006): 969–78, http://www.ncbi.nlm.nih.gov/pubmed/16741195.

129. L. Arab and A. Ang, "A Cross Sectional Study of the Association between Walnut Consumption and Cognitive Function among Adult U.S. Populations Represented in NHANES," *Journal of Nutrition, Health, and Aging* 19, no. 3 (2015): 284–290, http://link.springer.com/article/10.1007/s12603-014-0569-2#.

130. Ibid.

131. Elizabeth Gough-Gordon, "Vitamin B_3 May Reduce Recurrence of Some Skin Cancers in High-Risk Patients," *MPR*, May 14, 2015, http://www.empr.com/news/vitamin-b3-may-reduce-recurrence-of-some-skin-cancers-in-high-risk-patients/article/414669/?DCMP=EMC-MPR_DailyDose_cp&CPN=flecmpr, steld, xolderm&hmSubId=&hmEmail=LUGbza6izzVZv4gxnvu2QsU5jYgc1zdl0&dl=0&spMailingID=11390997&spUserID=MTgxMDI1NzYzMjY4S0&spJobID=540951443&spReportId=NTQwOTUxNDQzS0.

132. Ross D. Whitehead, Daniel Re, Dengke Xiao, et al., "You Are What You Eat: Within-Subject Increases in Fruit and Vegetable Consumption Confer Beneficial Skin-Color Changes," *PLOS One*, March 7, 2012, http://journals.plos.org/plosone/article?id=10.1371/journal.pone.0032988.

133. Li-Shu Wang and Gary D. Stoner, "Anthocyanins and Their Role in Cancer Prevention," *Cancer Letters* 269, no. 2 (2008): 281–90, http://www.cancerletters.info/article/S0304-3835(08)00396-0/abstract.

134. Won Jin Ho, Michael S. Simon, Vedat O. Yildiz, et al., "Antioxidant Micronutrients and the Risk of Renal Cell Carcinoma in the Women's Health Initiative Cohort," *Cancer*, first published online October 9, 2014, http://onlinelibrary.wiley.com/doi/10.1002/cncr.29091/abstract?systemMessage=Wiley+Online+Library+will+be+disrupted+on+7th+March+from+10%3A00-13%3A00+GMT+%2805%3A00

-08%3A00+EST%29+for+essential+maintenance.++Apologies+for +the+inconvenience.

135. A. V. Rao and L. G. Rao, "Carotenoids and Human Health," *Pharmacological Res*earch 55, no. 3 (2007): 207–16, http://www.ncbi.nlm.nih.gov/pubmed/17349800; Julie A. Evans and Elizabeth J. Johnson, "The Role of Phytonutrients in Skin Health," *Nutrients* 2, no. 8 (2010): 903–28, http://www.ncbi.nlm.nih.gov/pmc/articles/PMC3257702/.

136. D. Esser, M. Mars, E. Oosterink, et al., "Dark Chocolate Consumption Improves Leukocyte Adhesion Factors and Vascular Function in Overweight Men," *FASEB Journal* 28, no. 3 (2013): 1464–1473, http://www.fasebj.org/content/28/3/1464.

137. Ulrike Heinrich, Karin Neukam, Hagen Tronnier, et al., "Long-Term Ingestion of High Flavonol Cocoa Provides Photoprotection against UV-Induced Erythema and Improves Skin Condition in Women," *Journal of Nutrition* 136, no. 6 (2006): 1565–1569, http://jn.nutrition.org/content/136/6/1565.full.

138. Andrew Weil, "Turmeric Health Benefits: Have a Happy New Year With Turmeric," *Huffington Post*, December 28, 2010, http://www.huffingtonpost.com/andrew-weil-md/turmeric-health-have-a-happy-new-year_b_798328.html.

139. R. L. Thangapazham, A. Sharma, R. K. Maheshwari, "Beneficial Role of Curcumin in Skin Diseases," *Advances in Experimental Medicine and Biology* 595 (2007): 343–57, http://www.ncbi.nlm.nih.gov/pubmed/17569219.

140. Maho Sumiyohsi and Yoshiyuki Kimura, "Effects of a Turmeric Extract (Curcuma Longa) on Chronic Ultraviolet B

Irradiation-Induced Skin Damage in Melanin-Possessing Hairless Mice," *Phytomedicine* 16, no. 12 (2009): 1137–1143, http://www.sciencedirect.com/science/article/pii/S0944711309001640.

141. Anna Baghdasaryan, Thierry Claudel, Astrid Kosters, et al., "Curcumin Improves Sclerosing Cholangitis in Mdr2-/- Mice by Inhibition of Cholangiocyte Inflammatory Response and Portal Myofibroblast Proliferation," *Gut*, no. 59 (2010): 521–530, http://gut.bmj.com/content/59/4/521.full.pdf.

142. Tess Brensing, "Reduction of Heterocyclic Amine Formation in Beef By Surface Application of Spices," KREx K State Research Exchange, Kansas State University, December 2011, https://krex.k-state.edu/dspace/bitstream/handle/2097/13120/TessBrensing2011.pdf?sequence=1.

143. B. B. Aggarwal, A. Kumar, A. C. Bharti, "Anticancer Potential of Curcumin: Preclinical and Clinical Studies," *Anticancer Research* 23, no. 1A (2003): 363–98, http://www.ncbi.nlm.nih.gov/pubmed/12680238.

144. Ibid.

145. Murali M. Yallapu, Diane M. Maher, Vasudha Sundram, et al., "Curcumin Induces Chemo/Radio-sensitization in Ovarian Cancer Cells and Curcumin Nanoparticles Inhibit Ovarian Cancer Cell Growth," *Journal of Ovarian Research*, no. 3 (2010): 11, http://www.ovarianresearch.com/content/3/1/11.

146. "Spice Up Your Memory: Just One Gram of Turmeric a Day Could Boost Memory," *ScienceDaily*, November 18, 2014, http://www.sciencedaily.com/releases/2014/11/141118110009.htm?utm_source=feedburner&utm_medium=email&utm_campaign=Feed

%3A+sciencedaily%2Ftop_news%2Ftop_health+%28ScienceDaily %3A+Top+Health+News%29.

147. M. Fiala, P. T. Liu, A. Espinosa-Jeffrey, et al., "Innate Immunity and Transcription of MGAT-III and Toll-Like Receptors in Alzheimer's Disease Patients Are Improved by Bisdemethoxycurcumin," *Proceedings of the National Academy of Science* USA 104, no. 31 (2007): 12849–54, http://www.ncbi.nlm.nih.gov/pmc/articles/PMC1937555/.

148. C. Baron-Menguy, A. Bocquet, A. L. Guihot, et al. "Effects of Red Wine Polyphenols on Postischemic Neovascularization Model in Rats: Low Doses Are Proangiogenic, High Doses Anti-Angiogenic," *FASEB Journal* 21, no. 13 (2007): 3511–21, http://www.eurekalert.org/pub_releases/2007-10/foas-cir102907.php.

149. Diana Ernst, "New Evidence on How Certain Foods Provide Protective Health Benefits," *MPR*, April 13, 2015, http://www.empr.com/news/new-evidence-on-how-certain-foods-provide-protective-health-benefits/article/408654/?DCMP=EMC-MPR_DailyDose_rd&CPN=flecmpr, steld, xolderm&hmSubId=&hmEmail=LUGbza6izzVZv4gxnvu2QsU5jYgc1zdl0&dl=0&spMailingID=11141060&spUserID=MzA3NTI4MTQwMjAS1&spJobID=520998351&spReportId=NTIwOTk4MzUxS0.

150. Harrison Wein, "How Resveratrol May Fight Aging," *NIH Research Matters*, National Institutes of Health, http://www.nih.gov/researchmatters/march2013/03252013resveratrol.htm.

151. Albert Sanchez, J. L. Reeser, H. S. Lau, et al., "Role of Sugars in Human Neutrophilic Phagocytosis," *American Journal of Clinical Nutrition* 26, no. 11 (1973): 1180–1184, http://ajcn.nutrition.org/content/26/11/1180.abstract.

152. "Could Using an Artificial Sweetener Lead to Weight Gain?," *News from Harvard Health*, Harvard Health Publications, December 2011, http://www.health.harvard.edu/press_releases/could-using-an-artificial-sweetener-lead-to-weight-gain.

153. "10 Lifestyle Steps to Help Your Acne," WebMD, http://www.webmd.com/skin-problems-and-treatments/acne/features/lifestyle.

154. David Tin Win, "Oleic Acid—the Anti-Breast Cancer Component in Olive Oil," *AU Journal of Technology* 9, no. 2 (2005): 75–78, http://www.journal.au.edu/au_techno/2005/oct05/vol9num2_article02.pdf.

155. E. Cho, D. Spiegelman, D. J. Hunter, "Premenopausal Fat Intake and Risk of Breast Cancer," *Journal of the National Cancer Institute* 95, no. 14:1079–85, http://www.ncbi.nlm.nih.gov/pubmed/12865454.

156. Cynthia Aranow, "Vitamin D and the Immune System," *Journal of Investigative Medicine* 59, no. 6 (2011): 881–886, http://www.ncbi.nlm.nih.gov/pmc/articles/PMC3166406/.

157. "Vitamin D Protects against Colorectal Cancer by Boosting the Immune System," Dana-Farber Cancer Institute Newsroom, January 15, 2015, http://www.dana-farber.org/Newsroom/News-Releases/Vitamin-D-protects-against-colorectal-cancer-by-boosting-the-immune-system.aspx.

159. David C. R. Kerr, David T. Zava, Walter T. Piper, et al., "Associations between Vitamin D Levels and Depressive Symptoms in Healthy Young Adult Women," Psychiatry Research, published online March 6, 2015, http://www.psy-journal.com/article/S0165-1781(15)00108-0/abstract.

160. Mercedes Clemente-Postigo, Araceli Munoz-Garach, Marta Serrano, et al., "Serum 25-Hydroxyvitamin D and Adipose Tissue Vitamin D Receptor Gene Expression: Relationship With Obesity and Type 2 Diabetes," *Journal of Clinical Endocrinology & Metabolism*, published online February 23, 2015, http://press.endocrine.org/doi/abs/10.1210/jc.2014-3016.

161. "Vitamin D Deficiency Linked More Closely to Diabetes than Obesity," Endocrine Society, February 23, 2015, https://www.endocrine.org/news-room/current-press-releases/vitamin-d-deficiency-linked-more-closely-to-diabetes-than-obesity.

162. Carlos A. Camargo, Jr., D. Ganmaa, Robert Sidbury, et al., "Randomized Trial of Vitamin D Supplementation for Winter-Related Atopic Dermatitis in Children," *Journal of Allergy and Clinical Immunology* 134, no. 4 (2014): 831–835.e1, http://www.jacionline.org/article/S0091-6749(14)01114-2/abstract.

163. C. S. Kim, T. Kawada, B. S. Kim, et al., "Capsaicin Exhibits Anti-Inflammatory Property by Inhibiting IkB-a Degradation in LPS-Stimulated Peritoneal Macrophages," *Cellular Signalling* 15, no. 3 (2003): 299–306, http://www.ncbi.nlm.nih.gov/pubmed/12531428.

164. "Hot Pepper Compound Could Help Hearts," American Chemical Society, March 27, 2012, http://www.acs.org/content/acs/en/pressroom/newsreleases/2012/march/hot-pepper-compound-could-help-hearts.html.

165. Jun Lv, Lu Qi, Canqing Yu, et al., "Consumption of Spicy Foods and Total and Cause Specific Mortality: Population Based Cohort Study," *BMJ* 351 (2015): h3942, http://www.bmj.com/content/351/bmj.h3942.

166. "Do Coffee Drinkers Live Longer?," *MPR*, November 17, 2015, http://www.empr.com/medical-news/reduced-mortality-risk-seen-for-coffee-drinkers/article/454508/?DCMP=EMC-MPR_DailyDose_cp&cpn=flecmpr%2csteld%2cxolderm&hmSubId=&hmEmail=LUGbza6izzVZv4gxnvu2QsU5jYgc1zdl0&NID=1700857323&dl=0&spMailingID=13019299&spUserID=MTgwMTYxMDE2MjI0S0&spJobID=661426675&spReportId=NjYxNDI2Njc1S0.

167. Brenda Goodman, "Study Links Coffee to Lower Liver Cancer Risk," *HealthDay*, April 9, 2014, http://consumer.healthday.com/vitamins-and-nutrition-information-27/caffeine-health-news-89/more-java-please-686666.html.

168. "More Coffee May Mean Less Endometrial Cancer Risk," *MPR*, February 6, 2015, http://www.empr.com/more-coffee-may-mean-less-endometrial-cancer-risk/article/396947/?DCMP=EMC-MPR_DailyDose_rd&CPN=flecmpr, steld, xolderm&hmSubId=&hmEmail=LUGbza6izzVZv4gxnvu2QsU5jYgc1zdl0&dl=0&spMailingID=10587262&spUserID=MzA3NTI4MTQwMjAS1&spJobID=480508601&spReportId=NDgwNTA4NjAxS0.

169. A. H. Rosendahl, C. M. Perks, L. Zeng, et al., "Caffeine and Caffeic Acid Inhibit Growth and Modify Estrogen Receptor (ER) and Insulin-Like Growth Factor I Receptor (IGF-IR) Levels in Human Breast Cancer," *Clinical Cancer Research* 21 (2015): 1877, http://clincancerres.aacrjournals.org/content/21/8/1877.

170. Erikka Loftfield, Neal D. Freedman, Barry I. Graubard, et al., "Coffee Drinking and Cutaneous Melanoma Risk in the NIH-AARP Diet and Health Study," *JNCI* 107, no. 2 (2015), http://jnci.oxfordjournals.org/content/107/2/dju421.

171. Mikaela Conley, "Coffee May Reduce the Risk of Heart Failure," *ABC News*, June 26, 2012, http://abcnews.go.com/Health/coffee-reduce-heart-failure-risk/story?id=16652479.

172. "Drinking up to Five Cups of Coffee a Day May Benefit the Arteries," *Medical News Today*, March 3, 2015, http://www.medicalnewstoday.com/articles/290201.php.

173. Krishna Ramanujan, "A Cup of Coffee May Keep Retinal Damage Away," *Cornell Chronicle*, Cornell University, April 28, 2014, http://www.news.cornell.edu/stories/2014/04/cup-coffee-day-may-keep-retinal-damage-away.

174. "New Evidence That Drinking Coffee May Reduce the Risk of Diabetes," *American Chemical Society News*, June 9, 2010, http://www.acs.org/content/acs/en/pressroom/presspacs/2010/acs-presspac-june-09-2010/new-evidence-that-drinking-coffee-may-reduce-the-risk-of-diabetes.html.

175. Michel Lucas, Fariba Mirzaei, An Pan, et al., "Coffee, Caffeine, and Risk of Depression among Women," *JAMA Internal Medicine* 171, no. 17 (2011): 1571–1578, http://archinte.jamanetwork.com/article.aspx?articleid=1105943.

176. "Can Coffee Reduce Your Risk of MS?," *ScienceDaily*, February 26, 2015, http://www.sciencedaily.com/releases/2015/02/150226163245.htm.

177. Anthony Rivas, "Drinking Coffee Can Lower Alzheimer's Risk by 20%, All It Takes Is 3 Cups a Day," *Medical Daily*, November 26, 2014, http://www.medicaldaily.com/drinking-coffee-can-lower-alzheimers-risk-20-all-it-takes-3-cups-day-312410.

178. M. H. Eskelinen and M. Kivipelto, "Caffeine as a Protective Factor in Dementia and Alzheimer's Disease," *Journal of Alzheimer's Disease* 20, Supplement 1 (2010): S167–74, http://www.ncbi.nlm.nih.gov/pubmed/20182054.

179. David S. Lopez, Run Wang, Konstantinos K. Tsilidis, et al., "Role of Caffeine Intake on Erectile Dysfunction in US Men: Results from NHANES 2001–2004," *PLOS One*, April 28, 2015, http://journals.plos.org/plosone/article?id=10.1371/journal.pone.0123547.

180. S. Higgins, C. Straight, and R. D. Lewis, "The Effects of Pre-Exercise Caffeinated-Coffee Ingestion on Endurance Performance: An Evidence-Based Review," *International Journal of Sport Nutrition and Exercise Metabolism*, November 16, 2015, http://www.ncbi.nlm.nih.gov/pubmed/26568580.

181. Michael Greger, "Isn't Regular Cocoa Powder Healthier Than Alkali-Processed 'Dutched' Cocoa?," *NutritionFacts.Org*, November 7, 2012, http://nutritionfacts.org/questions/is-regular-cocoa-powder-healthier-than-dutched/.

182. Sushovita Mukherjee, Mohammad Adnan Siddiqui, et al., "Epigallocatechin-3-Gallate Suppresses Proinflammatory Cytokines and Chemokines Induced by Toll-like Receptor 9 Agonists in Prostate Cancer Cells," *Journal of Inflammation Research*, June 17, 2014, http://www.ncbi.nlm.nih.gov/pmc/articles/PMC4070858/.

183. "Can Drinking Tea Reduce Fracture Risk in Older Women?," *Consultant 360*, October 16, 2015, http://www.consultant360.com/exclusives/can-drinking-tea-reduce-fractures-older-women.

184. "Tea and Cancer Prevention: Strengths and Limits of the Evidence," National Cancer Institute Fact Sheet, National Cancer Institute at the National Institutes of Health, http://www.cancer.gov/cancertopics/factsheet/prevention/tea.

185. "Link between Vitamin E, Exposure to Air Pollution," *ScienceDaily*, May 15, 2015, http://www.sciencedaily.com/releases/2015/05/150515001122.htm?utm_source=feedburner&utm_medium=email&utm_campaign=Feed%3A+sciencedaily%2Ftop_news%2Ftop_health+%28ScienceDaily%3A+Top+Health+News%29.

186. "Extra Vitamin E Protected Older Mice from Getting Common Type of Pneumonia," *ScienceDaily*, December 16, 2014, http://www.sciencedaily.com/releases/2014/12/141216100429.htm?utm_source=feedburner&utm_medium=email&utm_campaign=Feed%3A+sciencedaily%2Ftop_news%2Ftop_health+%28ScienceDaily%3A+Top+Health+News%29.

187. T. Tsujita, T. Shintani, and H. Sato, "α-Amylase Inhibitory Activity from Nut Seed Skin Polyphenols. 1. Purification and Characterization of Almond Seed Skin Polyphenols," *Journal of Agricultural and Food Chemistry* 61, no. 19 (2013): 4570–6, https://www.ncbi.nlm.nih.gov/pubmed?term=J.+Agric.+Food+Chem.+[Jour]+AND+61[volume]+AND+4570[page]+AND+2013[pdat]&cmd=detailssearch#.

188. Z. Liu, X. Lin, G. Huang, et al., "Prebiotic Effects of Almonds and Almond Skins on Intestinal Microbiota in Healthy Adult Humans," *Anaerobe* 26 (2014): 1–6, https://www.ncbi.nlm.nih.gov/pubmed?term=Anaerobe[Jour]+AND+26[volume]+AND+1[page]+AND+2014[pdat]&cmd=detailssearch.

189. Monika Katyal Sachdeva, Taruna Katyal, "Abatement of Detrimental Effects of Photoaging by Prunus Amygdalus Skin Extract," *International Journal of Current Pharmaceutical Research* 3, no. 1 (2011): 57–59, http://www.ijcpr.org/Issues/Vol3Issue1/266.pdf.

190. Sylvia Booth Hubbard, "Why Women Live Longer Than Men," *NewsMax Health,* June 8, 2015, http://www.newsmax.com/Health/Health-News/women-men-longevity-super-centenarians/2015/06/08/id/649386/.

191. Fangui Sun, Paola Sebastiani, Nicole Schupf, et al., "Extended Maternal Age at Birth of Last Child and Women's Longevity in the Long Life Family Study," *Menopause* 22, no. 1 (2015): 26–31, http://journals.lww.com/menopausejournal/Citation/2015/01000/Extended_maternal_age_at_birth_of_last_child_and.7.aspx.

192. Ben Dulken and Anne Brunet, "Stem Cell Aging and Sex: Are We Missing Something?," *Cell Stem Cell* (2015), http://cdn.coverstand.com/27799/259797/1a11d5c8d5d178074f1ad6467145f5ea36e6692f.1.pdf.

193. Shota Miyata, Yozo Oda, and Chika Matsuo, "Stimulatory Effect of Brazilian Propolis on Hair Growth through Proliferation of Keratinocytes in Mice," *Journal of Agricultural and Food Chemistry* 62, no. 49 (2014): 11854–11861, http://pubs.acs.org/doi/abs/10.1021/jf503184s.

Chapter 2: Cultivate Inner Peace and Spirituality

194. J. Kabat-Zinn, E. Wheeler, T. Light, et al., "Influence of a Mindfulness Meditation-Based Stress Reduction Intervention on Rates of Skin Clearing in Patients with Moderate to Severe Psoriasis Undergoing Phototherapy (UVB) and Photochemotherapy

(PUVA)," *Psychosomatic Medicine* 60, no. 5 (1998): 625–632, http://www.ncbi.nlm.nih.gov/pubmed/9773769.

195. "How Managing Stress May Help Your Psoriasis," Health, http://www.health.com/health/gallery/0,,20306771,00.html.

196. "Anti-InflammatoryDiet,"NationalPsoriasisFoundation,http://www.psoriasis.org/treating-psoriasis/complementary-and-alternative/diet-and-nutrition/anti-inflammatory-diet.

197. D. S. Krantz, K. S. Whittaker, and D. S. Sheps, "Psychosocial Risk Factors for Coronary artery Disease: Pathophysiologic Mechanisms," in R. Allan and J. Fisher, eds., *In Heart and Mind: Evolution of Cardiac Psychology* (Washington, DC: APA, 2011), 91–113.

198. "TheEffectsofStressontheBody,"June24,2014,http://www.webmd.com/balance/stress-management/effects-of-stress-on-your-body.

199. "Stress in America" survey, American Psychological Association, 2012.

200. Charles Bankhead, "Is Stress Taking a Toll on Our Skin?," *Medpage Today*, August 10, 2014, http://www.medpagetoday.com/MeetingCoverage/AAD/47139.

201. "Stress Effects," The American Institute of Stress, http://www.stress.org/stress-effects/.

202. "Stress, Depression and Antidepressant Treatment Options in Patients Suffering from Multiple Sclerosis," *Current Pharmaceutical Design* 18, no. 36 (2012): 5837–5845, http://www.ncbi.nlm.nih.gov/pubmed/22681164.

203. B. Haque, K. M. Rahman and A. Hoque, "Precipitating and Relieving Factors of Migraine Versus Tension Type Headache," *BMC Neurology* 12 (2012): 82, http://www.ncbi.nlm.nih.gov/pmc/articles/PMC3503560/.

204. B. G. Schwartz, W. J. French, G. S. Mayeda, et al., "Emotional Stressors Trigger Cardiovascular Events," *International Journal of Clinical Practice* 66, no. 7 (2012): 631–9, http://www.ncbi.nlm.nih.gov/pubmed/22698415; A. Steptoe and M. Kivimaki, "Stress and Cardiovascular Disease," *Nature Reviews Cardiology* 9, no. 6 (2012): 360–70, http://www.ncbi.nlm.nih.gov/pubmed/22473079.

205. "Stress May Play a Key Role in the Development of Type II Diabetes in Obese Black Women, U.S. Researchers Say," *HealthDay News*, March 5, 2009, http://bit.ly/1xTMbku.

206. M. L. Harris, D. Loxton, D. W. Sibbritt, and J. E. Byles, "The Influence of Perceived Stress on the Onset of Arthritis in Women: Findings from the Australian Longitudinal Study on Women's Health," *Annals of Behavioral Medicine* 46, no. 1 (2013): 9–18, http://www.ncbi.nlm.nih.gov/pubmed/23436274.

207. Ann M. Hemmerle, James P. Herman, and Kim B. Seroogy, "Stress, Depression, and Parkinson's Disease," *Experimental Neurology* 233, no. 1 (2012): 79–86, http://www.ncbi.nlm.nih.gov/pmc/articles/PMC3268878/.

208. S. Cohen, D. Janicki-Deverts, and G. E. Miller, "Psychological Stress and Disease," *JAMA* 298, no. 14 (2007): 1685–7, http://www.ncbi.nlm.nih.gov/pubmed/17925521.

209. Susan J. Broughton, Matthew D. W. Piper, Tomoatsu Ikeya, et al., "Longer Lifespan, Altered Metabolism, and Stress Resistance in

Drosophila from Ablation of Cells Making Insulin-Like Ligands," *PNAS: Proceedings of the National Academy of Sciences* 102, no. 8 (2005): 3105–3110, http://www.pnas.org/content/102/8/3105.full; "Metabolism: Does Stress Really Shorten Your Life?," National Institute on Aging, November 2011, http://www.nia.nih.gov/health/publication/biology-aging/metabolism-does-stress-really-shorten-your-life.

210. Ibid.

211. "Are Telomeres the Key to Aging and Cancer?" Learn.Genetics, http://learn.genetics.utah.edu/content/chromosomes/telomeres/.

212. "Mediterranean Diet Linked to Longer Life," *ScienceDaily*, December 3, 2014, http://www.sciencedaily.com/releases/2014/12/141203084255.htm?utm_source=feedburner&utm_medium=email&utm_campaign=Feed%3A+sciencedaily%2Ftop_news%2Ftop_health+%28ScienceDaily%3A+Top+Health+News%29.

213. "Telomere Extension Turns Back Aging Clock in Cultured Human Cells, Study Finds," *ScienceDaily*, January 23, 2015, http://www.sciencedaily.com/releases/2015/01/150123102539.htm?utm_source=feedburner&utm_medium=email&utm_campaign=Feed%3A+sciencedaily%2Ftop_news%2Ftop_health+%28ScienceDaily%3A+Top+Health+News%29.

214. Michelle Bragazzi, "Telomere Length May Be Associated With Melanoma Risk," *OncoTherapy Network*, November 6, 2014, http://www.oncotherapynetwork.com/skin-cancer-melanoma-targets/telomere-length-may-be-associated-melanoma-risk.

215. Ibid.

216. Paula Martinez and Maria A. Blasco, "Replicating through Telomeres: A Means to an End," *Trends in Biochemical Sciences*, July 14, 2015, http://www.cell.com/trends/biochemical-sciences/abstract/S0968-0004(15)00114-0?_returnURL=http%3A%2F%2Flinkinghub.elsevier.com%2Fretrieve%2Fpii%2FS0968000415001140%3Fshowall%3Dtrue.

217. Marta Crous-Bou, Teresa F. Fung, Jennifer Prescott, et al., "Mediterranean Diet and Telomere Length in Nurses' Health Study: Population Based Cohort Study," *BMJ* 349 (2014): g6674, http://www.bmj.com/content/349/bmj.g6674.

218. S. Duraimani, R. H. Schneider, O. S. Randall, et al., "Effects of Lifestyle Modification on Telomerase Gene Expression in Hypertensive Patients: A Pilot Trial of Stress Reduction and Health Education Programs in African Americans," *PLOS ONE* 10, no. 11 (2015), http://journals.plos.org/plosone/article?id=10.1371/journal.pone.0142689.

219. Ying Chen and John Lyga, "Brain-Skin Connection: Stress, Inflammation, and Skin Aging," *Inflammation and Allergy Drug Targets* 13, no. 3 (2014): 177–190, http://www.eurekaselect.com/122325/article.

220. Ibid.

221. Ibid.

222. M. Lebwohl and L. G. Herrmann, "Impaired Skin Barrier Function in Dermatologic Disease and Repair with Moisturization," *Cutis* 76, no. 6 (2005): 7–12, http://www.ncbi.nlm.nih.gov/pubmed/16869176; N. Muizzuddin, M. S. Matsui, K. D. Marenus, et al., "Impact of Stress of Marital Dissolution on Skin Barrier

Recovery: Tape Stripping and Measurement of Trans-Epidermal Water Loss (TEWL)," *Skin Research and Technology* 9, no. 1 (2003): 34–38, http://www.ncbi.nlm.nih.gov/pubmed/12535282.

223. Jean-Philippe Gouin and Janice K. Kiecolt-Glaser, "The Impact of Psychological Stress on Wound Healing: Methods and Mechanisms," *Immunology and Allergy Clinics of North America* 31, no. 1 (2011): 81–93, http://www.ncbi.nlm.nih.gov/pmc/articles/PMC3052954/.

224. Ying Chen and John Lyga, "Brain-Skin Connection: Stress, Inflammation, and Skin Aging," *Inflammation and Allergy Drug Targets* 13, no. 3 (2014): 177–190, http://www.eurekaselect.com/122325/article; Petra C. Arck, Andrzej Slominski, Theoharis C. Theoharides, et al., "Neuroimmunology of Stress: Skin Takes Center Stage," *Journal of Investigative Dermatology* 126, no. 8 (2006): 1697–1704, http://www.ncbi.nlm.nih.gov/pmc/articles/PMC2232898/.

225. "What Is Alopecia Areata? What Causes Alopecia Areata?," *Medical News Today*, August 19, 2014, http://www.medicalnewstoday.com/articles/70956.php.

226. J. Parker, S. L. Klein, M. K. McClintock, et al., "Chronic Stress Accelerates Ultraviolet-Induced Cutaneous Carcinogenesis," *Journal of the American Academy of Dermatology* 51, no. 6 (2004): 919–22, http://www.ncbi.nlm.nih.gov/pubmed/15583583; Alison N. Saul, Tatiana M. Oberyszyn, Christine Daugherty, et al., "Chronic Stress and Susceptibility to Skin Cancer," *Journal of the National Cancer Institute* 97, no. 23 (2005): 1760–67, http://www.ncbi.nlm.nih.gov/pmc/articles/PMC3422720/.

227. Ilya Petrou, "Pollution, Stress Take Toll on Skin Aging," *Dermatology Times*, February 1, 2014, http://dermatologytimes.

modernmedicine.com/dermatology-times/content/tags/anti-aging/pollution-stress-take-toll-skin-aging?page=full.

228. P. Oyetakin-White, B. Koo, M. Matsui, et al., "Effects of Sleep Quality on Skin Aging and Function," *Journal of Investigative Dermatology* (2013) : S126–S126, http://www.nature.com/jid/journal/v133/n1s/full/jid201399a.html.

229. "Vitamin C: Stress Buster," *Psychology Today*, April 25, 2003, http://www.psychologytoday.com/articles/200304/vitamin-c-stress-buster.

230. Russell Blaylock, "Stress Depletes Vitamin C," *Newsmax Health*, January 7, 2015, http://www.newsmaxhealth.com/RussellBlaylockMD/vitamin-C-stress-antioxidant-anemia/2015/01/07/id/617099/?ns_mail_uid=80858862&ns_mail_job=1602913_01102015&s=al&dkt_nbr=q4uthzra.

231. Erica M. Schulte, Nicole M. Avena, and Ashley N. Gearhardt, "Which Foods May Be Addictive? The Roles of Processing, Fat Content, and Glycemic Load," *PLOS One*, February 18, 2015, http://journals.plos.org/plosone/article?id=10.1371/journal.pone.0117959.

232. "Chemicals in Cigarette Smoke," Centers for Disease Control and Prevention, http://www.cdc.gov/tobacco/data_statistics/sgr/2010/consumer_booklet/chemicals_smoke/index.htm.

233. Ibid.

234. C. Kennedy, M. T. Bastiaens, C. D. Bajdik, et al., "Effect of Smoking and Sun on the Aging Skin," *Journal of Investigative*

Dermatology 120, no. 4 (2003): 548–54, http://www.ncbi.nlm.nih.gov/pubmed/12648216.

235. "Health Effects of Secondhand Smoke," Centers for Disease Control and Prevention, http://www.cdc.gov/tobacco/data_statistics/fact_sheets/secondhand_smoke/health_effects/.

236. Gideon St. Helen, Peyton Jacob III, Margaret Peng, et al., "Intake of Toxic and Carcinogenic Volatile Organic Compounds from Secondhand Smoke in Motor Vehicles," *Cancer Epidemiology, Biomarkers & Prevention* 23 (2014): 2774, http://cebp.aacrjournals.org/content/23/12/2774.

237. G. Ferrante, M. Simoni, F. Cibella, et al, "Third-hand Smoke Exposure and Health Hazards in Children," *Monaldi Archives for Chest Disease* 79, no. 1 (2013): 38–43, http://www.ncbi.nlm.nih.gov/pubmed/23741945.

238. Nancy L. Sin, Jennifer E. Graham-Engleland, Anthony D. Ong, et al., "Affective Reactivity to Daily Stressors Is Associated With Elevated Inflammation," *Health Psychology*, June 1, 2015, http://psycnet.apa.org/?&fa=main.doiLanding&doi=10.1037/hea0000240.

239. Suzanne C. Segerstrom and Gregory E. Miller, "Psychological Stress and the Human Immune System: A Meta-Analytic Study of 30 Years of Inquiry," *Psychological Bulletin* 130, no. 4 (2004): 601–630, http://www.ncbi.nlm.nih.gov/pmc/articles/PMC1361287/.

240. Ed Diener and Micaela Y. Chan, "Happy People Live Longer: Subjective Well-Being Contributes to Health and Longevity," *Applied Psychology: Health and Well-Being* 3, no. 1 (2011): 1–43, http://onlinelibrary.wiley.com/doi/10.1111/j.1758-0854.2010.01045.x/full.

241. Sheldon Cohen, Denise Janicki-Deverts, Ronald B. Turner, et al., "Does Hugging Provide Stress-Buffering Social Support? A Study of Susceptibility to Upper Respiratory Infection and Illness," *Psychological Science*, December 19, 2014, published online before print, http://pss.sagepub.com/content/early/2014/12/17/0956797614559284.

242. Claire Carter, "Sex Is the Secret to Looking Younger, Claims Researcher," *Telegraph*, July 5, 2013, http://www.telegraph.co.uk/lifestyle/10161279/Sex-is-the-secret-to-looking-younger-claims-researcher.html.

243. Sara Rimer, "Happiness and Health," *Harvard School of Public Health News*, Winter 2011, http://www.hsph.harvard.edu/news/magazine/happiness-stress-heart-disease/; "How Happiness Affects Your Health," March 27, 2013, http://abcnews.go.com/blogs/health/2013/03/27/how-happiness-affects-your-health/.

244. Erik J. Giltay, Johanna M. Geleijnse, Frans G. Zitman, et al., "Dispositional Optimism and All-Cause and Cardiovascular Mortality in a Prospective Cohort of Elderly Dutch Men and Women," *JAMA Psychiatry* 61, no. 11 (2004): 1126–1135, http://archpsyc.jamanetwork.com/article.aspx?articleid=482087.

245. Diana Yates, "Study: Happiness Improves Health and Lengthens Life," *Illinois News Bureau*, March 1, 2011, http://news.illinois.edu/NEWS/11/0301happy_EdDiener.html.

246. Jane Collingwood, "Study Probes How Emotions Affect the Immune System," *PsychCentral*, May 22, 2014, http://psychcentral.com/news/2014/05/22/study-probes-how-emotions-affect-immune-system/70192.html.

247. "What Is Mindfulness Meditation?," Mindfulness-Based Stress Reduction in Central Pennsylvania, http://meditationscience.weebly.com/what-is-mindfulness-meditation.html.

248. "Meditation Programs for Psychological Stress and Well-Being: A Systemic Review and Meta-Analysis," *JAMA Internal Medicine* 174, no. 3 (2014): 357–368, http://archinte.jamanetwork.com/article.aspx?articleid=1809754.

249. Tom Scheve, "Is There a Link Between Exercise and Happiness?," How Stuff Works, http://science.howstuffworks.com/life/exercise-happiness.htm.

250. Elizabeth A. Hoge, Eric Bui, and Luana Marques, "Randomized Controlled Trial of Mindfulness Meditation for Generalized Anxiety Disorder: Effects on Anxiety and Stress Reactivity," *Journal of Clinical Psychology* 74, no. 8 (2013): 786–792, http://www.ncbi.nlm.nih.gov/pmc/articles/PMC3772979/.

251. R. P. Brown and P. L. Gerbarg, "Yoga Breathing, Meditation, and Longevity," *Annals of the New York Academy of Sciences* 1172 (2009): 54–62, http://www.pubfacts.com/detail/19735248/Protection-throughout-the-life-span:-the-psychoneuroimmunologic-impact-of-Indo-Tibetan-meditative-an.

252. "Diaphragmatic Breathing," Cleveland Clinic Diseases & Conditions, http://my.clevelandclinic.org/health/diseases_conditions/hic_Understanding_COPD/hic_Pulmonary_Rehabilitation_Is_it_for_You/hic_Diaphragmatic_Breathing.

253. Ibid.

254. Sharita Forest, "Optimistic People Have Healthier Hearts, Study Finds," Illinois News Bureau, January 8, 2015, https://news.illinois.edu/news/15/0108optimism_rosalbahernandez.html.

255. S. L. Warber, S. Ingerman, V. L. Moura, et al., "Healing the Heart: A Randomized Pilot Study of a Spiritual Retreat for Depression in Acute Coronary Syndrome Patients," *Explore* 7, no. 4 (2011): 222–33, http://www.explorejournal.com/article/S1550-8307(11)00099-1/abstract.

256. Allen R. McConnell, Christina M. Brown, Tonya M. Shoda, et al., "Friends With Benefits: On the Positive Consequences of Pet Ownership," *Journal of Personality and Social Psychology* 101, no. 6 (2011): 1239–1252, http://psycnet.apa.org/psycinfo/2011-13783-001/.

257. Allen R. McConnell, "Friends with Benefits: Pets Make Us Happier, Healthier," *Psychology Today*, July 11, 2011, http://www.psychologytoday.com/blog/the-social-self/201107/friends-benefits-pets-make-us-happier-healthier.

258. "Why Stress Causes People to Overeat," *Harvard Mental Health Letter*, Harvard Health Publications, February 2012, http://www.health.harvard.edu/newsletters/harvard_mental_health_letter/2012/february/why-stress-causes-people-to-overeat.

259. E. Epel, R. Lapidus, B. McEwen, et al., "Stress May Add Bite to Appetite in Women: A Laboratory Study of Stress-Induced Cortisol and Eating Behavior," *Psychoneuroendocrinology* 26, no. 1 (2001): 37–49, www.ncbi.nlm.nih.gov/pubmed/11070333.

260. Jennifer O'Brien, "Comfort Food Cravings May Be Body's Attempt to Put Brake on Chronic Stress," University of California San Francisco News Center, September 10, 2003, http://www.ucsf.edu/news/2003/09/4682/comfort-food-cravings-may-be-bodys-attempt-put-brake-chronic-stress.

261. Erica M. Shulte, Nicole M. Avena, and Ashley N. Gearhardt, "Which Foods May Be Addictive? The Roles of Processing, Fat Content, and Glycemic Load," *PLOS One*, February 18, 2015, http://journals.plos.org/plosone/article?id=10.1371/journal.pone.0117959.

262. A. E. Moyer, J. Rodin, C. M. Grilo, N. Cummings, et al., "Stress-Induced Cortisol Respose and Fat Distribution in Women," *Obesity Research* 2, no. 3 (1994): 255–62, http://www.ncbi.nlm.nih.gov/pubmed/16353426.

263. Ananya Mandal, "Obesity and Skin Problems," *News Medical*, http://www.news-medical.net/health/Obesity-and-skin-problems.aspx.

264. Erin L. Olivo, "Protection throughout the Life Span: The Psychoneuroimmunologic Impact of Indo-Tibetan Meditative and Yogic Practices," *Annals of the New York Academy of Sciences* 1172 (2009): 163–71, http://www.pubfacts.com/detail/19735248/Protection-throughout-the-life-span:-the-psychoneuroimmunologic-impact-of-Indo-Tibetan-meditative-an.

265. J. Kiecolt-Glaser and R. Glaser, "The Stress and Health Research Program," The Ohio State University Institute for Behavioral Medicine Research, http://pni.osumc.edu.

266. "Acupuncture: What You Need to Know," National Center for Complementary and Alternative Medicine, http://nccam.nih.gov/health/acupuncture/introduction; Andrew J. Vickers, Angel M. Cronin, Alexandra C. Maschino, et al., "Acupuncture for Chronic Pain," *JAMA Internal Medicine* 72, no. 19 (2012): 1444–1453, http://archinte.jamanetwork.com/article.aspx?articleid=1357513.

267. B. Khamba, M. Aucoin, M. Lytle, et al., "Efficacy of Acupuncture Treatment of Sexual Dysfunction Secondary to Antidepressants," *Journal of Alternative and Complementary Medicine* 19, no. 11 (2013): 862–9, http://www.ncbi.nlm.nih.gov/pubmed/23790229.

268. "Acupuncture Shows Promise in Improving Rates of Pregnancy Following IVF," National Center for Complementary and Alternative Medicine, http://nccam.nih.gov/research/results/spotlight/020808.htm.

269. S. Hu, R. Stritzel, A. Chandler, et al., "P6 Acupressure Reduces Symptoms of Vection-Induced Motion Sickness," *Aviation, Space, and Environmental Medicine* 66, no. 7 (1995): 631–4, http://www.ncbi.nlm.nih.gov/pubmed/7575310.

270. "Dysmenorrhea: Principal Proposed Natural Treatments," NYU Langone Medical Center, http://www.med.nyu.edu/content?ChunkIID=21602.

271. Ian D. Bier, Jeffrey Wilson, Pat Studt, et al., "Auricular Acupuncture, Education, and Smoking Cessation: A Randomized, Sham-Controlled Trial," *American Journal of Public Health* 92, no. 10 (2002): 1642–1647, http://www.ncbi.nlm.nih.gov/pmc/articles/PMC1447300/.

272. "Oregon Study Confirms Health Benefits of Cobblestone Walking for Older Adults," *ScienceDaily*, June 30, 2005, http://www.sciencedaily.com/releases/2005/06/050630055256.htm.

273. "Acupuncture for Eczema & Skin Disorders," Pacific College of Oriental Medicine, http://www.pacificcollege.edu/news/blog/2015/01/16/acupuncture-eczema-skin-disorders.

274. Chelsea Ma and Raja K. Sivamani, "Acupuncture as a Treatment Modality in Dermatology: A Systematic Review," *Journal of Alternative and Complementary Medicine*, June 26, 2015, http://online.liebertpub.com/doi/abs/10.1089/acm.2014.0274?journalCode=acm.

275. Rose Adams, Barb White, and Cynthia Beckett, "The Effects of Massage Therapy on Pain Management in the Acute Care Setting," *International Journal of Therapeutic Massage & Bodywork* 3, no. 1 (2010): 4–11, http://www.ncbi.nlm.nih.gov/pmc/articles/PMC3091428/.

276. Emily Caldwell, "Study: Massaging Muscles Facilitates Recovery After Exercise," *The Ohio State University Research News*, August 12, 2008, http://researchnews.osu.edu/archive/compload.htm.

277. Jason Brummit, "The Role of Massage in Sports Performance and Rehabilitation: Current Evidence and Future Direction," *North American Journal of Sports Physical Therapy* 3, no. 1 (2008): 7–21, http://www.ncbi.nlm.nih.gov/pmc/articles/PMC2953308/.

278. Ibid.

279. L. Lindgren, S. Rundgren, O. Winso, et al., "Physiological Responses to Touch Massage in Healthy Volunteers," *Autonomic Neuroscience* 158, no. 1–2 (2010): 105–110, http://www.autonomic-neuroscience.com/article/S1566-0702%2810%2900127-X/pdf.

280. Ibid.

281. A. D. Kaye, A. J. Kaye, J. Swinford, et al., "The Effect of Deep-Tissue Massage Therapy on Blood Pressure and Heart Rate," *Journal of Alternative and Complementary Medicine* 14, no. 2 (2008): 125–8, http://www.ncbi.nlm.nih.gov/pubmed/18315516.

282. Jeanne Galatzer-Levy, "Massage Therapy Improves Circulation, Eases Muscle Soreness," University of Illinois at Chicago News Center, April 15, 2014, http://news.uic.edu/massage-therapy-improves-circulation-alleviates-muscle-soreness.

283. Bruno Chikly, "Lymph Drainage Therapy: An Effective Complement to Breast Care," *Massagetherapy.com*, http://www.massagetherapy.com/articles/index.php/article_id/207/Lymph-Drainage-Therapy.

284. A. Billhuit, C. Lindholm, Ronny Gunnarsson, et al., "The Effect of Massage on Immune Function and Stress in Women with Breast Cancer—a Randomized Controlled Trial," *Autonomic Neuroscience* 150, no. 1–2 (2009): 111–115, http://www.autonomicneuroscience.com/article/S1566-0702%2809%2900085-X/abstract.

285. J. Stringer, R. Swindell, and M. Dennis, "Massage in Patients Undergoing Intensive Chemotherapy Reduces Serum Cortisol and Prolactin," *Psycho-Oncology* 17, no. 10 (2008): 1024–31, http://www.ncbi.nlm.nih.gov/pubmed/18300336.

286. Daniel Goleman, "The Experience of Touch: Research Points to a Critical Role," *New York Times*, February 2, 1988, http://www.nytimes.com/1988/02/02/science/the-experience-of-touch-research-points-to-a-critical-role.html; "Massage," University of Maryland Medical Center, http://umm.edu/health/medical/altmed/treatment/massage.

287. "Osteopathy," University of Maryland Medical Center, October 13, 2011, http://umm.edu/health/medical/altmed/treatment/osteopathy.

288. B. F. Degenhardt, N. A. Darmani, J. C. Johnson, et al., "Role of Osteopathic Manipulative Treatment in Altering Pain Biomarkers: A Pilot Study," *Journal of the American Osteopathic Association* 107, no. 9 (2007): 387–400, http://www.ncbi.nlm.nih.gov/pubmed/17908831.

289. Joanna Broder, "Low Back Pain: Osteopathic Manual Therapy Appears to Help," *Medscape Multispecialty Medical News*, March 18, 2013, http://www.medscape.com/viewarticle/781005.

290. Richard John Clark, "Depression, Anxiety and Positive Outlook Amongst Patients Presenting to an Osteopathic Training Clinic: A Prospective Survey," Unitec Institute of Technology, 2010, http://unitec.researchbank.ac.nz/bitstream/handle/10652/1509/Richard%20Clarke%20MOst.pdf?sequence=1.

291. Rosemary E. Anderson and Caryn Sensiscal, "A Comparison of Selected Osteopathic Treatment and Relaxation for Tension-Type Headaches," *Headache* 46, no. 8 (2006): 1273–80, http://www.researchgate.net/publication/6847241_A_comparison_of_selected_osteopathic_treatment_and_relaxation_for_tension-type_headaches.

292. D. R. Noll, J. H. Shores, R. G. Gamber, et al., "Benefits of Osteopathic Manipulative Treatment for Hospitalized Elderly Patients with Pneumonia," *Journal of the American Osteopathic Association* 100, no. 12 (2000): 776–782, http://www.ncbi.nlm.nih.gov/pubmed/11213665.

293. J. Hibler, Jessie Perkins, David Eland, et al., "Osteopathic Manipulative Medicine for Inflammatory Skin Diseases," *Journal of the American Osteopathic College of Dermatology* 31:11–13, http://c.

ymcdn.com/sites/www.aocd.org/resource/resmgr/jaocd/jaocd-vol31.pdf.

294. Victoria Houghton, "Defining the DO," *Dermatology World*, June 2015, 28–33.

295. "Tai Chi," National Center for Complementary and Alternative Medicine, http://nccam.nih.gov/health/taichi.

296. "Tai Chi Helps Parkinson's Patients with Balance and Fall Prevention," National Institute of Neurological Disorders and Stroke, May 10, 2012, http://www.ninds.nih.gov/news_and_events/news_articles/Li_TaiChi_and_PD.htm.

297. P. M. Wayne, D. P. Kiel, D. E. Krebs, et al., "The Effects of Tai Chi on Bone Mineral Density in Postmenopausal Women: A Systematic Review," *Archives of Physical Medicine and Rehabilitation* 88, no. 5 (2007): 673–80, http://www.ncbi.nlm.nih.gov/pubmed/17466739.

298. C. Lan, S. Y. Chen, M. K. Wong, et al., "Tai Chi Training for Patients with Coronary Heart Disease," *Medicine and Sport Science* 52 (2008): 182–94, http://www.ncbi.nlm.nih.gov/pubmed/18487898.

299. "Tai Chi Boosts Immunity to Shingles Virus in Older Adults, NIH-Sponsored Study Reports," *NIH News*, April 6, 2007, http://www.ncbi.nlm.nih.gov/pubmed/18487898.

300. "The Effects of Tai Chi on Depression, Anxiety, and Psychological Well-Being: A Systematic Review and Analysis," *International Journal of Behavioral Medicine* 21, no. 4 (2014): 605–17, http://www.ncbi.nlm.nih.gov/pubmed/24078491.

301. "Tai Chi," National Center for Complementary and Alternative Medicine, http://nccam.nih.gov/health/taichi.

302. Ned Hartfiel, Jon Havenhand, Sat Bir Khalsa, et al., "The Effectiveness of Yoga for the Improvement of Well Being and Resilience to Stress in the Workplace," *Scandinavian Journal of Work, Environment & Health*, 2011, http://science.naturalnews.com/2011/835887_The_effectiveness_of_yoga_for_the_improvement_of_well_being.html.

303. Samantha Olson, "Yoga Can Reduce Risk of Heart Disease; Practice These Types of Yoga for Better Health," *Medical Daily*, December 16, 2014, http://www.medicaldaily.com/yoga-can-reduce-risk-heart-disease-practice-these-types-yoga-better-heart-health-314532.

304. M. S. Garfinkel, A. Singhal, W. A. Katz, et al., "Yoga-Based Intervention for Carpal Tunnel Syndrome: A Randomized Trial," *JAMA* 280, no. 18 (1998): 1601–3, http://www.ncbi.nlm.nih.gov/pubmed/9820263.

305. Demeke Mekonnen and Andualem Mossie, "Clinical Effects of Yoga on Asthmatic Patients: A Preliminary Clinical Trial," *Ethiopian Journal of Health Sciences* 20, no. 2 (2010): 107–112, http://www.ncbi.nlm.nih.gov/pmc/articles/PMC3275836/.

306. H. E. Tilbrook, H. Cox, C. E. Hewitt, et al., "Yoga for Chronic Back Pain: A Randomized Trial," *Annals of Internal Medicine* 155, no. 9 (2011): 569–78, http://www.ncbi.nlm.nih.gov/pubmed/22041945.

307. N. R. Okonta, "Does Yoga Therapy Reduce Blood Pressure in Patients With Hypertension: An Integrative Review," *Holistic*

Nursing Practice 26, no. 3 (2012): 137–41, http://www.ncbi.nlm.nih.gov/pubmed/22517349.

308. R. F. Afonso, H. Hachul, E. H. Kozasa, et al., "Yoga Decreases Insomnia in Postmenopausal Women: A Randomized Clinical Trial," *Menopause* 19, no. 2 (2012): 186–93, http://www.ncbi.nlm.nih.gov/pubmed/22048261.

309. Steffany Haaz and Susan J. Bartlett, "Yoga for Arthritis: A Scoping Review," *Rheumatic Disease Clinics of North America* 37, no. 1 (2011): 33–46, http://www.ncbi.nlm.nih.gov/pmc/articles/PMC3026480/.

310. Badr Aljasir, Maggie Bryson, and Bandar Al-shehri, "Yoga Practice for the Management of Type II Diabetes Mellitus in Adults: A Systematic Review," *Evidence-Based Complementary and Alternative Medicine* 7, no. 4 (2010): 399–408, http://www.ncbi.nlm.nih.gov/pmc/articles/PMC2892348/.

311. S. B. Khalsa, "Treatment of Chronic Insomnia with Yoga: A Preliminary Study with Sleep-Wake Diaries," *Applied Psychophysiology and Biofeedback* 29, no. 4 (2004): 269–78, http://www.ncbi.nlm.nih.gov/pubmed/15707256.

312. Ananda Balayogi Bhavanani and Zeena Sanjay, "Effect of Yoga on Subclinical Hypothyroidism: A Case Report," *Yoga Mimamsa* 43, no. 2 (2012): 102–107, http://www.researchgate.net/publication/237075972_Effect_of_yoga_on_subclinical_hypothyroidism_a_case_report.

313. L. Kuttner, C. T. Chambers, J. Hardial, et al., "A Randomized Trial of Yoga for Adolescents with Irritable Bowel Syndrome," *Pain*

Research & Management 11, no. 4 (2006): 217–23, http://www.ncbi.nlm.nih.gov/pubmed/17149454?dopt=AbstractPlus.

314. Paul Leher, Richard E. Carr, Alexander Smetankine, et al., "Respiratory Sinus Arrhythmia Versus Neck/Trapezius EMG and Incentive Inspirometry Biofeedback for Asthma: A Pilot Study," *Applied Psychology and Biofeedback* 22, no. 2 (1997): 95–109, http://scholar.google.com/scholar_url?url=http://www.researchgate.net/profile/Erik_Peper/publication/259184685_1997_RSA_and_Asthma_Lehrer_et_al/links/00b7d52a3a535c7f44000000.pdf&hl=en&sa=X&scisig=AAGBfm02kkMHT7LPFbtpp4Tvx4AY_xIeWQ&nossl=1&oi=scholarr.

315. A. Dobbin, J. Dobbin, S. C. Ross, et al., "Randomised Controlled Trial of Brief Intervention with Biofeedback and Hypnotherapy in Patients with Refractory Irritable Bowel Syndrome," *Journal of the Royal College of Physicians of Edinburgh* 43, no. 1 (2013): 15–23, http://www.ncbi.nlm.nih.gov/pubmed/23516685.

316. W. J. Mullally, K. Hall, and R. Goldstein, "Efficacy of Biofeedback in the Treatment of Migraine and Tension Type Headaches," *Pain Physician* 12, no. 6 (2009): 1005–11, http://www.ncbi.nlm.nih.gov/pubmed/19935987.

317. G. Tan, J. Thornby, D. C. Hammond, et al., "Meta-analysis of EEG Biofeedback in Treating Epilepsy," *Clinical EEG and Neuroscience* 40, no. 3 (2009): 173–9, http://www.ncbi.nlm.nih.gov/pubmed/19715180.

318. David Schardt, "Managing Menopause," *Nutrition Action Healthletter*, July/August 2004, https://www.cspinet.org/nah/07_04/managing_menopause.pdf.

319. P. Hauri, "Treating Psychophysiologic Insomnia with Biofeedback," *Archives of General Psychiatry* 38, no. 7 (1981): 752–8, http://www.ncbi.nlm.nih.gov/pubmed/7247638.

320. Judith A. Turner and C. Richard Chapman, "Psychological Interventions for Chronic Pain: A Critical Review. I. Relaxation Training and Biofeedback," *Pain*, January 1982, 1–21, http://www.sciencedirect.com/science/article/pii/0304395982901671.

321. D. E. Yocum, R. Hodes, W. R. Sundstrom, et al., "Use of Biofeedback Training in Treatment of Raynaud's Disease and Phenomenon," *Journal of Rheumatology* 12, no. 1 (1985): 90–3, http://www.ncbi.nlm.nih.gov/pubmed/3981523.

322. L. Kranitz and P. Lehrer, "Biofeedback Applications in the Treatment of Cardiovascular Diseases," *Cardiology in Review* 12, no. 3 (2004): 177–81, http://www.ncbi.nlm.nih.gov/pubmed/15078588.

323. M. E. D. Jarrett, A. V. Emmanuel, C. J. Vaizey, et al., "Behavioural Therapy (Biofeedback) for Solitary Rectal Ulcer Syndrome Improves Symptoms and Mucosal Blood Flow," *Gut* 53, no. 3 (2004): 368–370, http://www.ncbi.nlm.nih.gov/pmc/articles/PMC1773992/.

324. Alan Brauer, "Biofeedback and Anxiety," *Psychiatric Times*, February 1, 1999, http://www.psychiatrictimes.com/articles/biofeedback-and-anxiety.

325. T. G. Burish and R. A. Jenkins, "Effectiveness of Biofeedback and Relaxation Training in Reducing the Side Effects of Cancer Chemotherapy," *Health Psychology* 11, no. 1 (1992): 17–23, http://www.ncbi.nlm.nih.gov/pubmed/1559530.

326. A. McGrady, B. K. Bailey, M. P. Good, "Controlled Study of Biofeedback-Assisted Relaxation in Type I Diabetes," *Diabetes Care* 14, no. 5 (1991): 360–5, http://www.ncbi.nlm.nih.gov/pubmed/2060447.

327. "Research Findings Using Guided Imagery for Hypertension," Academy for Guided Imagery, August 2006, http://acadgi.com/whatisguidedimagery/page25/page26/page34/page34.html.

328. Jason C. Ong, Shauna L. Shapiro, and Rachel Manber, "Combining Mindfulness Meditation with Cognitive-Behavior Therapy for Insomnia," *Behavior Therapy* 39, no. 2 (2008): 171–82, http://www.ncbi.nlm.nih.gov/pmc/articles/PMC3052789/.

329. J. L. Apostolo and K. Colcaba, "The Effects of Guided Imagery on Comfort, Depression, Anxiety, and Stress of Psychiatric Inpatients with Depressive Disorders," *Archives of Psychiatric Nursing* 23, no. 6 (2009): 403–11, http://www.ncbi.nlm.nih.gov/pubmed/19926022.

330. "Research Findings Using Guided Imagery for Irritable Bowel Syndrome," Academy for Guided Imagery, August 2006, http://www.academyforguidedimagery.com/research/medical/irritable/.

331. C. Lahmann, M. Nickel, T. Schuster, et al., "Functional Relaxation and Guided Imagery as Complementary Therapy in Asthma: A Randomized Controlled Clinical Trial," *Psychotherapy and Psychosomatics* 78 (2009): 233–239, https://www.google.com/webhp?sourceid=chrome-instant&ion=1&espv=2&ie=UTF-8#q=guided+imagery+and+allergies+and+asthma+research.

332. S. Karagozoglu, F. Tekyasar, and F. A. Yilmaz, "Effects of Music Therapy and Guided Visual Imagery on Chemotherapy-Induced

Anxiety and Nausea-Vomiting," *Journal of Clinical Nursing* 22, no. 1–2 (2013): 39–50, http://www.ncbi.nlm.nih.gov/pubmed/23134272.

333. Laurie F. Kubes, "CE: Imagery for Self-Healing and Integrative Nursing Practice," *American Journal of Nursing* 115, no. 11 (2015): 36–43, http://journals.lww.com/ajnonline/Fulltext/2015/11000/CE___Imagery_for_Self_Healing_and_Integrative.22.aspx.

334. C. Papantonio, "Alternative Medicine and Wound Healing," *Ostonomy/Wound Management* 44, no. 4 (1998): 44–50, http://www.ncbi.nlm.nih.gov/pubmed/9611606.

335. Yi-Yuan Tang, Qilin Lu, Ming Fan, et al., "Mechanisms of White Matter Changes Induced by Meditation," *PNAS* 109, no. 26 (2012): 10570–10574, http://www.pnas.org/content/109/26/10570.abstract.

336. Marc Kaufman, "Meditation Gives Brain a Charge, Study Finds," *Washington Post,* January 3, 2005, A05, http://www.washingtonpost.com/wp-dyn/articles/A43006-2005Jan2.html.

337. Ellen Luders, Nicolas Cherbuin, and Florian Kurth, "Forever Young(er): Potential Age-Defying Effects of Long-Term Meditation on Gray Matter Atrophy," *Frontiers in Psychology,* January 21, 2015, http://journal.frontiersin.org/journal/10.3389/fpsyg.2014.01551/abstract.

338. Britta K. Höizel, James Carmody, Mark Vangel, et al., "Mindfulness Practice Leads to Increases in Regional Brain Gray Matter Density," *Psychiatry Research Neuroimaging* 191, no. 1 (2011): 36–43, http://www.psyn-journal.com/article/S0925-4927(10)00288-X/abstract.

339. Alex Hankey, "Studies of Advanced Stages of Meditation in the Tibetan Buddhist and Vedic Traditions. I: A Comparison of General Changes," *Evidence-Based Complementary and Alternative Medicine* 3, no. 4 (2006): 513–521, http://www.ncbi.nlm.nih.gov/pmc/articles/PMC1697747/.

340. "Meditation May Reduce Death, Heart Attack, and Stroke in Heart Patients," American Heart Association Newsroom, November 13, 2012, http://newsroom.heart.org/news/meditation-may-reduce-death-heart-240647.

341. A. B. Newberg, N. Wintering, D. S. Khalsa, et al., "Meditation Effects on Cognitive Function and Cerebral Blood flow in Subjects with Memory Loss: A Preliminary Study," *Journal of Alzheimer's Disease* 20, no. 2 (2010): 517–526, http://www.ncbi.nlm.nih.gov/pubmed/20164557#.

342. J. Kabat-Zinn, L. Lipworth, and R. Burney, "The Clinical Use of Mindfulness Meditation for the Self-Regulation of Chronic Pain," *Journal of Behavioral Medicine* 8, no. 2 (1985): 163–90, http://www.ncbi.nlm.nih.gov/pubmed/3897551.

343. Elizabeth A. Hoge, Eric Bui, Luana Marques, et al., "Randomized Controlled Trial of Mindfulness Meditation for Generalized Anxiety Disorder: Effects on Anxiety and Stress Reactivity," *Journal of Clinical Psychiatry* 74, no. 8 (2013): 786–792, http://www.ncbi.nlm.nih.gov/pmc/articles/PMC3772979/.

344. E. H. Kozasa, L. H. Tanaka, C. Monson, et al., "The Effects of Meditation-Based Interventions on the Treatment of Fibromyalgia," *Current Pain and Headache Reports* 16, no. 5 (2012): 383–7, http://www.ncbi.nlm.nih.gov/pubmed/22717699.

345. K. A. Zernicke, T. S. Campbell, P. K. Blustein, et al., "Mindfulness-Based Stress Reduction for the Treatment of Irritable Bowel Syndrome Symptoms: A Randomized Wait-List Controlled Trial," *International Journal of Behavioral Medicine* 20, no. 3 (2013): 385–96, http://www.ncbi.nlm.nih.gov/pubmed/22618308.

346. "The Science of Meditation for Mind & Body Health," McLean Meditation Institute, http://www.sedonameditation.com/meditation-research.html; Jeanie Lerche Davis, "Meditation Balances the Body's Systems," WedMD, http://www.webmd.com/balance/features/transcendental-meditation.

347. F. Zeidan, J. A. Grant, C. A. Brown, et al., "Mindful Meditation-Related Pain Relief: Evidence for Unique Brain Mechanisms in the Regulation of Pain," *Neuroscience Letters* 520, no. 2 (2012): 165–73, http://www.ncbi.nlm.nih.gov/pubmed/22487846.

348. Brian Krans, "Study: Meditation's Effects Similar to Pills for Depression," *HealthlineNews*, January 6, 2014, http://www.healthline.com/health-news/mental-meditation-as-effective-as-medication-for-depression-010614; "Meditation Effective in Treating Anxiety, Depression, Hopkins Research Suggests," HUB: Johns Hopkins News Network, January 8, 2014, http://hub.jhu.edu/2014/01/08/meditate-to-reduce-depression.

349. Dessa Bergen-Cico, Kyle Possemato, and Wilfred Pigeon, "Reductions in Cortisol Associated with Primary Care Brief Mindfulness Program for Veterans with PTSD," *Medical Care* 52 (December 2014): S25–S31, http://journals.lww.com/lww-medicalcare/Fulltext/2014/12001/Reductions_in_Cortisol_Associated_With_Primary.8.aspx.

350. W. C. Chen, H. Chu, R. B. Lu, et al., "Efficacy of Progressive Muscle Relaxation Training in Reducing Anxiety in Patients with

Acute Schizophrenia," *Journal of Clinical Nursing* 18, no. 15 (2009): 2187–96, http://www.ncbi.nlm.nih.gov/pubmed/19583651.

351. C. Nickel, C. Kettler, M. Muehlbacher, et al., "Effect of Progressive Muscle Relaxation in Adolescent Female Bronchial Asthma Patients: A Randomized, Double-Blind, Controlled Study," *Journal of Psychosomatic Research* 59, no. 6 (2005): 393–8, http://www.ncbi.nlm.nih.gov/pubmed/16310021.

352. Alexandru Bogdan Vasile, Robert Balazsi, Viorel Lupu, et al., "Treating Primary Insomnia: A Comparative Study of Self-Help Methods and Progressive Muscle Relaxation," *Journal of Evidence-Based Psychotherapies* 9, no. 1 (2009), http://jebp.psychotherapy.ro/vol-ix-no-1/treating-primary-insomnia-a-comparative-study-of-self-help-methods-and-progressive-muscle-relaxation/.

353. S. Sheu, B. L. Irvin, H. S. Lin, et al., "Effects of Progressive Muscle Relaxation on Blood Pressure and Psychosocial Status for Clients with Essential Hypertension in Taiwan," *Holistic Nursing Practice* 17, no. 1 (2003): 41–7, http://www.ncbi.nlm.nih.gov/pubmed/12597674.

354. Mark P. Jensen, Joseph Barber, Joan M. Romano, et al., "A Comparison of Self-Hypnosis Versus Progressive Muscle Relaxation in Patients with Multiple Sclerosis and Chronic Pain," *International Journal of Clinical and Experimental Hypnosis* 57, no. 2 (2009): 198–221, http://www.ncbi.nlm.nih.gov/pmc/articles/PMC2758639/.

355. Adam Burke, "Comparing Individual Preferences for Four Meditation Techniques: Zen, Vipassana (Mindfulness), Qigong, and Mantra," *Explore: The Journal of Science and Healing* 8, no. 4 (2012): 237–242, http://www.explorejournal.com/article/S1550-8307%2812%2900077-8/abstract.

356. "Animal Therapy Reduces Anxiety, Loneliness Symptoms in College Students," *Georgia State University News*, October 21, 2014, http://news.gsu.edu/2014/10/21/animal-therapy-reduces-anxiety-loneliness-symptoms-college-students/.

357. Andrea Beetz, Kerstin Uvnas-Moberg, Henri Julius, et al., "Psychosocial and Psychophysiological Effects of Human-Animal Interactions: The Possible Role of Oxytocin," *Frontiers in Psychology*, published online July 9, 2012, http://www.ncbi.nlm.nih.gov/pmc/articles/PMC3408111/.

358. Al Jones, "Zoetis-Funded Study Supports Beneficial Link between Animal Therapy and Cancer Patients," *MLive*, January 17, 2015, http://www.mlive.com/business/west-michigan/index.ssf/2015/01/zoetis-funded_study_supports_b.html.

359. "Get Healthy, Get a Dog: The Health Benefits of Canine Companionship," *Harvard Medical School Special Health Report*, http://www.health.harvard.edu/special-health-reports/get-healthy-get-a-dog.

360. Maria Beatriz Silva Borges, Maria Jose da Silva Werneck, Maria de Lourdes da Silva, et al., "Therapeutic Effects of a Horse Riding Simulator in Children with Cerebral Palsy," *Arquivos de Neuro-Psiquiatria* 69, no. 5 (2011): 799–804, http://www.scielo.br/scielo.php?script=sci_arttext&pid=S0004-282X2011000600014&lng=en&nrm=iso&tlng=en.

361. Sima Ash, "Animals Rescue Children with Autism, ADHD, and Dyslexia," *NaturalHealth365*, April 7, 2013, http://www.naturalhealth365.com/autism_news/animals_therapy.html.

362. Lindsay Wilson, "Animal-Assisted Therapy," *Exceptional Children*, http://faculty.frostburg.edu/mbradley/EC/animalassistedtherapy.html.

363. Alex Stone, "Smell Turns Up in Unexpected Places," *New York Times*, October 13, 2014, http://www.nytimes.com/2014/10/14/science/smell-turns-up-in-unexpected-places.html?ref=health&_r=0.

364. Mary Margaret Chappell, "Aromatherapy for Pain Relief," Arthritis Foundation, http://www.arthritistoday.org/arthritis-treatment/natural-and-alternative-treatments/remedies-and-therapies/aromatherapy-pain-relief.php?utm_source=MBSnewsletter&utm_medium=email&utm_term=aromatherapy&utm_content=body1&utm_campaign=Jan15.

365. H. Moradkhani, E. Sargsyan, H. Bibak, et al., "*Melissa Officinalis* L., a Valuable Medicine Plant: A Review," *Journal of Medicinal Plants Research* 4, no. 25 (2010): 2753–2759, http://www.academicjournals.org/article/article1380713061_Moradkhani%20et%20al.pdf.

366. Ibid.

367. Christa Sinadinos, "Herbs at a Glance," The Northwest School for Botanical Studies, http://www.herbaleducation.net/herbs-glance.

368. "The Human Brain: Renew-Relieve Stress," The Franklin Institute, http://learn.fi.edu/learn/brain/relieve.html.

369. Heather L. Stuckey and Jeremy Nobel, "The Connection Between Art, Healing, and Public Health: A Review of Current Literature," *American Journal of Public Health* 100, no. 2 (2010): 254–263, http://ajph.aphapublications.org/doi/abs/10.2105/AJPH.2008.156497.

370. C. Crawford, C. Lee, J. Bingham, et al., "Sensory Art therapies for the Self-Management of Chronic Pain Symptoms," *Pain Medicine*, Supplement 1 (2014): S66–75, http://www.ncbi.nlm.nih.gov/pubmed/24734861.

371. Heather L. Stuckey and Jeremy Nobel, "The Connection Between Art, Healing, and Public Health: A Review of Current Literature," *American Journal of Public Health* 100, no. 2 (2010): 254–263, http://ajph.aphapublications.org/doi/abs/10.2105/AJPH.2008.156497.

372. Bree Chancellor, Angel Duncan, and Anjan Chatterjee, "Art Therapy for Alzheimer's Disease and Other Dementias," *Journal of Alzheimer's Disease* 39 (2014): 1–11, http://ccn.upenn.edu/chatterjee/anjan_pdfs/Chancellor_ArtTherapy_AD_JAD.pdf.

373. Jennifer E. Stellar, Neha John-Henderson, Craig L. Anderson, et al., "Positive Affect and Markers of Inflammation: Discrete Positive Emotions Predict Lower Levels of Inflammatory Cytokines," *Emotion*, January 19, 2015, http://psycnet.apa.org/?&fa=main.doiLanding&doi=10.1037/emo0000033.

374. Eleanor McKenzie, "The Reiki Bible: The Definitive Guide to Healing with Energy," Sterling, September 1, 2009.

375. Diane Wind Wardell and Kathryn F. Weymouth, "Review of Studies of Healing Touch," *Journal of Nursing Scholarship* 36, no. 2 (2004): 147–154, http://tigger.uic.edu/~darcovic/htreview.pdf.

376. Alam Khan, Mahpara Safdar, Mohammad Muzaffar Ali Khan, et al., "Cinnamon Improves Glucose and Lipids of People with Type 2 Diabetes," *Diabetes Care* 26, no. 12 (2003): 3215–3218, http://care.diabetesjournals.org/content/26/12/3215.abstract.

377. Min Long, Shasha Tao, Montserrat Rojo de la Vega, et al., "Nrf2-Dependent Suppression of Azoxymethane/Dextran Sulfate Sodium–Induced Colon Carcinogenesis by the Cinnamon-Derived Dietary Factor Cinnamaldehyde," *Cancer Prevention Research* 8 (May 2015): 444, http://cancerpreventionresearch.aacrjournals.org/content/8/5/444.

378. Yusra Al Dhaheri, Samir Attoub, Kholoud Arafat, et al., "Anti-Metastatic and Anti-Tumor Growth Effects of Origanummajorana on Highly Metastatic Human Breast Cancer Cells: Inhibition of NFκB Signaling and Reduction of Nitric Oxide Production," *PLOS One*, July 10, 2013, http://journals.plos.org/plosone/article?id=10.1371/journal.pone.00688.

379. J. J. Johnson, "Carnosol: A Promising Anti-Cancer and Anti-Inflammatory Agent," *Cancer Letters* 305, no. 1 (2011): 1–7, http://www.ncbi.nlm.nih.gov/pubmed/21382660.

380. "Compound Found in Rosemary Protects against Macular Degeneration in Laboratory Model," *ScienceDaily*, November 27, 2012, http://www.sciencedaily.com/releases/2012/11/121127154205.htm.

381. Vivian Tullio, Narcisa Mandras, Valeria Allizond, et al., "Positive Interaction of Thyme (Red) Essential Oil with Human Polymorphonuclear Granulocytes in Eradicating Intracellular *Candida albicans*," *Planta Medica* 78, no. 15 (2012): 1633–1635, https://www.thieme-connect.de/products/ejournals/abstract/10.1055/s-0032-1315153.

382. "Thymus Mastichina: Chemical Constituents and Their Anti-Cancer Activity," *Natural Product Communications* 7, no. 11 (2012): 1491–4, http://www.ncbi.nlm.nih.gov/pubmed/23285814.

383. B. B. Aggarwal, A. Kumar, and A. C. Bharti, "Anticancer Potential of Curcumin: Preclinical and Clinical Studies," *Anticancer Research* 23, no. 1A (2003): 363–98, http://www.ncbi.nlm.nih.gov/pubmed/12680238.

384. "Spice Up Your Memory: Just One Gram of Turmeric a Day Could Boost Memory," *ScienceDaily*, November 18, 2014, http://www.sciencedaily.com/releases/2014/11/141118110009.htm?utm_source=feedburner&utm_medium=email&utm_campaign=Feed%3A+sciencedaily%2Ftop_news%2Ftop_health+%28ScienceDaily%3A+Top+Health+News%29.

385. M. Fiala, P. T. Liu, A. Espinosa-Jeffrey, et al., "Innate Immunity and Transcription of MGAT-III and Toll-Like Receptors in Alzheimer's Disease Patients are Improved by Bisdemethoxycurcumin," *Proceedings of the National Academy of Science* USA 104, no. 31 (2007): 12849–54, http://www.ncbi.nlm.nih.gov/pmc/articles/PMC1937555/.

386. Yang Liu and Marcia A. Petrini, "Effects of Music Therapy on Pain, Anxiety, and Vital Signs in Patients After Thoracic Surgery," *Complementary Therapies in Medicine* 23, no. 5 (2015): 714–718, http://www.complementarytherapiesinmedicine.com/article/S0965-2299%2815%2900126-0/fulltext.

387. "New Study Confirms Listening to Music during Surgery Reduces Pain and Anxiety," *Queen Mary University of London News*, August 13, 2015, http://www.qmul.ac.uk/media/news/items/smd/160783.html.

388. Güler Balci Alparslan, Burcu Babadag, Ayse Ozkaraman, et al., "Effects of Music on Pain in Patients with Fibromyalgia," *Clinical*

Rheumatology, August 6, 2015, http://link.springer.com/article/10.1007%2Fs10067-015-3046-3.

389. Shelby R. Lies and Andrew Y. Zhang, "Prospective Randomized Study of the Effect of Music on the Efficiency of Surgical Closures," *Aesthetic Surgery Journal* 35, no. 7 (2015): 858–863, http://asj.oxfordjournals.org/content/35/7/858.

390. Q. Li, K. Morimoto, A. Nakadai, et al., "Forest Bathing Enhances Human Natural Killer Activity and Expression of Anti-Cancer Proteins," *International Journal of Immunopathology and Pharmacology* 20, 2 Supplement 2 (2007): 3–8, http://www.ncbi.nlm.nih.gov/pubmed/17903349.

391. Richard M. Ryan and Marylène Gagné, "Vitalizing Effects of Being Outdoors and in Nature," *Journal of Environmental Psychology* 30, no. 2 (2010): 159–168, http://www.sciencedirect.com/science/article/pii/S0272494409000838.

392. "Taking a Walk May Lead to More Creativity than Sitting, Study Finds," American Psychological Association, April 24, 2014, http://www.apa.org/news/press/releases/2014/04/creativity-walk.aspx.

393. Rob Jordan, "Stanford Researchers Find Mental Health Prescription: Nature," *Stanford News*, June 30, 2015, http://news.stanford.edu/news/2015/june/hiking-mental-health-063015.html.

394. "Glancing at a Grassy Green Roof Significantly Boosts Concentration," *Melbourne Newsroom*, May 25, 2015, http://newsroom.melbourne.edu/news/glancing-grassy-green-roof-significantly-boosts-concentration.

395. Rebecca A. Clay, "Green Is Good for You," *Monitor on Psychology* 32, no. 4 (2001): 40, http://www.apa.org/monitor/apr01/greengood.aspx.

396. Yuna L. Ferguson and Kennon M. Sheldon, "Trying to Be Happier Really Can Work: Two Experimental Studies," *Journal of Positive Psychology* 8, no. 1 (2013), http://www.tandfonline.com/doi/abs/10.1080/17439760.2012.747000?journalCode=rpos20.

397. Amy Westervelt, "Forgive to Live: New Research Shows Forgiveness is Good for the Heart," *Good,* August 25, 2012, http://magazine.good.is/articles/forgive-to-live-new-research-shows-forgiveness-is-good-for-the-heart.

398. Karen Kaplan, "'Purpose in Life' Can Help Reduce Medical Costs," *Seattle Times,* November 3, 2014, http://seattletimes.com/html/nationworld/2024946289_healthpurposexml.html.

399. Elisabeth Kübler-Ross, *Death: The Final Stage of Growth,* (Scribner, 1997), as seen in Wayne Dyer, *I Can See Clearly Now,* (Hay House, 2014), 261.

400. Elizabeth Svoboda, "Hard-Wired for Giving," *Wall Street Journal,* August, 31, 2013, http://www.wsj.com/articles/SB10001424127887324009304579041231971683854.

Chapter 3: Rethink Your Exercise Strategy

401. M. Pratt, C. A. Macera, and G. J. Wang, "Higher Direct Medical Costs Associated with Physical Inactivity," *Physician and SportsMedicine* 28 (2000): 63–70, http://www.ncbi.nlm.nih.gov/pubmed/20086598.

402. Trevor C. Nordin, Aaron J. Done, and Tinna Traustadottir, "Acute Exercise Increases Resistance to Oxidative Stress in Young, but

Not Older Adults," *AGE* 36 (2014): 9727, http://www.ncbi.nlm.nih.gov/pubmed/25380675.

403. I. Holme and S. A. Anderssen, "Increases in Physical Activity Is as Important as Smoking Cessation for Reduction in Total Mortality in Elderly Men: 12 Years of Follow-Up of the Oslo II Study," *British Journal of Sports Medicine* 49, no. 11 (2015): 743–748, http://bjsm.bmj.com/content/49/11/743.

404. Susan R. Barry, "How to Grow New Neurons in Your Brain," *Psychology Today*, January 16, 2011, https://www.psychologytoday.com/blog/eyes-the-brain/201101/how-grow-new-neurons-in-your-brain.

405. Heidi Godman, "Regular Exercise Changes the Brain to Improve Memory, Thinking Skills," *Harvard Health Publications*, April 9, 2014, http://www.health.harvard.edu/blog/regular-exercise-changes-brain-improve-memory-thinking-skills-201404097110.

406. Jun-Ming Zhang and Jianxiong An, "Cytokines, Inflammation, and Pain," *International Anesthesiology Clinics* 45, no. 2 (2007): 27–37, http://www.ncbi.nlm.nih.gov/pmc/articles/PMC2785020/.

407. Ibid.

408. Look AHEAD Research Group, "Reduction in Weight and Cardiovascular Disease Risk Factors in Individuals with Type 2 Diabetes: One-Year Results of the Look AHEAD Trial," *Diabetes Care* 30, no. 6 (2007): 1374–1383, http://www.ncbi.nlm.nih.gov/pmc/articles/PMC2665929/.

409. "Estrogen & Breast Cancer Risk: Factors of Exposure," Cornell University Program on Breast Cancer and Environmental Risk

Factors, July 2002, http://envirocancer.cornell.edu/factsheet/general/fs10.estrogen.cfm.

410. Gretchen Reynolds, "Phys Ed: Does Exercise Boost Immunity?," *New York Times.com*, October 14, 2009, http://well.blogs.nytimes.com/2009/10/14/phys-ed-does-exercise-boost-immunity/?_r=0.

411. H.J. Dennison, C. Cooper, A.A. Sayer, et al., "Prevention and Optimal Management of Sarcopenia: A Review of Combined Exercise and Nutrition Interventions to Improve Muscle Outcomes in Older People," *Clinical Interventions in Aging* 10 (2015): 859–869, http://www.dovepress.com/prevention-and-optimal-management-of-sarcopenia-a-review-of-combined-e-peer-reviewed-article-CIA.

412. Lynette L. Craft, Frank M. Perna, "The Benefits of Exercise for the Clinically Depressed," *Primary Care Companion Journal of Clinical Psychiatry* 6, no. 3 (2004): 104–11, http://www.ncbi.nlm.nih.gov/pmc/articles/PMC474733/.

413. Jonathan Myers, "Exercise and Cardiovascular Health," *Circulation* 107 (2003): e2–e5, http://circ.ahajournals.org/content/107/1/e2.full.

414. "How Does Exercise Help Those with Chronic Insomnia?," National Sleep Foundation, http://sleepfoundation.org/ask-the-expert/how-does-exercise-help-those-chronic-insomnia.

415. Miranda E. G. Armstrong, Jane Green, Gillian K. Reeves, et al., "Frequent Physical Activity May Not Reduce Vascular Disease Risk as Much as Moderate Activity: Large Prospective Study of UK Women," *Circulation* 131 (2015): 721–729, 10.1161/CIRCULATIONAHA.114.010296.

416. "Walking an Extra Two Minutes Each Hour May Offset Hazards of Sitting Too Long," University of Utah Healthcare, April 30, 2015, http://healthcare.utah.edu/publicaffairs/news/2015/04/04-30-15_short_walks_offset_hazards_of_sitting_too_long.php.

417. W.J. Crinnion, "Sauna as a Valuable Clinical Tool for Cardiovascular, Autoimmune, Toxicant-Induced and Other Chronic Health Problems," *Alternative Medicine Review* 16, no. 3 (2011): 215–225, http://www.altmedrev.com/publications/16/3/215.pdf.

418. Gretchen Reynolds, "Younger Skin through Exercise," *nytimes.com*, April 16, 2014, http://well.blogs.nytimes.com/2014/04/16/younger-skin-through-exercise/?_r=0.

419. Marshall Hagins, Wendy Moore, and Andrew Rundle, "Does Practicing Hatha Yoga Satisfy Recommendations for Intensity of Physical Activity Which Improves and Maintains Health and Cardiovascular Fitness?," *BMC Complementary and Alternative Medicine* 7 (2007): 40, http://www.biomedcentral.com/1472-6882/7/40.

420. A. Ross and S. Thomas, "The Health Benefits of Yoga and Exercise: a Review of Comparison Studies," *Journal of Alternative and Complementary Medicine* 16, no. 1 (2010): 3–12, http://www.ncbi.nlm.nih.gov/pubmed/20105062.

421. "Yoga for Health," National Center for Complementary and Alternative Health, https://nccih.nih.gov/health/yoga/introduction.htm.

422. "Yoga and Chronic Pain Have Opposite Effects on Brain Gray Matter," *Newswise*, May 15, 2015, http://www.newswise.com/articles/view/634072/?sc=mwhn.

Chapter 4: Get the Sleep You Need

423. "The Benefits of Walking: Walking Toward a Healthier You," The American Heart Association, http://www.startwalkingnow.org/whystart_benefits_walking.jsp.

424. "Insufficient Sleep Is a Public Health Epidemic," Centers for Disease Control and Prevention, http://www.cdc.gov/features/dssleep/index.html#References.

425. "Centenarian Secrets and Longevity Science," *CentenarianSecrets.Blogspot.com*, June 4, 2008, http://centenariansecrets.blogspot.com/2008/06/httpwww.html; Eiko Uezu, Kazuhiko Taira, Hideki Tanaka, et al., "Survey of Sleep-Health and Lifestyle of the Elderly in Okinawa," *Psychiatry and Clinical Neurosciences* 54 (2000): 311–313, http://onlinelibrary.wiley.com/store/10.1046/j.1440-1819.2000.00692.x/asset/j.1440-1819.2000.00692.x.pdf;jsessionid=927A3C895E34F82D3EB4AEB337181EDC.f04t04?v=1&t=iazk1uft&s=f34632c87df13a9d1b233a81d45615eba84303ee.

426. "CDC: 9 Million Americans Use Prescription Sleeping Pills," *DailyNews*, August 30, 2013, http://www.nydailynews.com/life-style/health/cdc-9-million-americans-sleeping-pills-article-1.1441778.

427. "Over-the-Counter Sleep Aids Linked to Dementia," *Medical News Today*, June 12, 2015, http://www.medicalnewstoday.com/articles/288546.php.

428. "Alzheimer's Linked to Sleeping Pills and Anti-Anxiety Drugs," *Time.com*, September 10, 2014, http://time.com/3313927/alzheimers-linked-to-sleeping-pills-and-anti-anxiety-drugs/.

429. Neil B. Kavey, "Why Do We Need Sleep So Much?," *NBCNews.com*, http://www.nbcnews.com/id/3076707/ns/technology_and_science-science/t/why-do-we-need-so-much-sleep/.

430. Jonathan Cedernaes, Megan E. Osler, Sarah Voisin, et al., "Acute Sleep Loss Induces Tissue-Specific Epigenetic and Transcriptional Alterations to Circadian Clock Genes in Men," *Journal of Clinical Endocrinology & Metabolism*, July 13, 2015, http://press.endocrine.org/doi/10.1210/JC.2015-2284.

431. Tara Haelle, "Poor Quality Sleep May Be Linked to a Shrinking Brain," *HealthDay*, September 3, 2014, http://consumer.healthday.com/senior-citizen-information-31/misc-aging-news-10/poor-quality-sleep-may-be-linked-to-shrinking-brain-691359.html.

432. J. Cedernaes, F.H. Rangtell, E.K. Axelsson, et al., "Short Sleep Makes Declarative Memories Vulnerable to Stress in Humans," *Sleep*, June 22, 2015, http://www.ncbi.nlm.nih.gov/pubmed/26158890.

433. Björn Rasch and Jan Born, "About Sleep's Role in Memory," *Physiological Reviews* 93, no. 2 (2013): 681–766, http://www.ncbi.nlm.nih.gov/pmc/articles/PMC3768102/; "Nothing Beats a Good Night's Sleep for Helping People Absorb New Information, New Research Reveals," *ScienceDaily*, http://www.sciencedaily.com/releases/2015/04/150417085218.htm?utm_source=feedburner&utm_medium=email&utm_campaign=Feed%3A+sciencedaily%2Ftop_news%2Ftop_health+%28ScienceDaily%3A+Top+Health+News%29.

434. "Sleep, Learning, and Memory," *Healthy Sleep*, Division of Sleep Medicine at Harvard Medical School, December 18, 2007, http://healthysleep.med.harvard.edu/healthy/matters/benefits-of-sleep/learning-memory.

435. Ibid.

436. "Poor Sleep Associated with Increased Risk of Heart Attack and Stroke," European Society of Cardiology, June 15, 2015, http://www.escardio.org/The-ESC/Press-Office/Press-releases/Last-5-years/Poor-sleep-associated-with-increased-risk-of-heart-attack-and-stroke.

437. H. Oginska and J. Pokorski, "Fatigue and Mood Correlates of Sleep Length in Three Age-Social Groups: School Children, Students, and Employees," *Chronobiology International* 26, no. 6 (2006): 1317–28, http://www.ncbi.nlm.nih.gov/pubmed/17190716.

438. Torbjorn Akerstedt, Johanna Garefelt, Anne Richter, et al., "Work and Sleep—a Prospective Study of Psychosocial Work Factors, Physical Work Factors, and Work Scheduling," *Sleep* 38, no. 7 (2015), http://www.journalsleep.org/ViewAbstract.aspx?pid=30081.

439. D. F. Dinges, F. Pack, K. Williams, et al., "Cumulative Sleepiness, Mood Disturbance, and Psychomotor Vigilance Performance Decrements during a Week of Sleep Restricted to 4–5 Hours Per Night," *Sleep* 20, no. 4 (1997): 267–277, http://www.ncbi.nlm.nih.gov/pubmed/9231952.

440. "Losing 30 Minutes of Sleep Per Day May Promote Weight Gain and Adversely Affect Blood Sugar Control," *Newswise.com*, March 5, 2015, http://www.newswise.com/articles/view/630723/?sc=mwhn.

441. Sanjay R. Patel, Atul Malhotra, David. P. White, et al., "Association between Reduced Sleep and Weight Gain in Women," *American Journal of Epidemiology* 164, no. 10 (2006): 947–954, http://aje.oxfordjournals.org/content/164/10/947.full; Donald Hensrud, "Is Too Little Sleep a Cause of Weight Gain?," *MayoClinic.Org*,

http://www.mayoclinic.org/healthy-lifestyle/adult-health/expert-answers/sleep-and-weight-gain/faq-20058198.

442. Nanci Hellmich, "How Sleep Loss Leads to Significant Weight Gain," *USA Today*, July 20, 2014, http://www.usatoday.com/story/news/nation/2014/07/20/sleep-loss-weight-gain/7507503/.

443. Rachel R. Markwald, Edward L. Melanson, Mark R. Smith, et al., "Impact of Insufficient Sleep on Total Daily Energy Expenditure, Food Intake, and Weight Gain," *Proceedings of the National Academy of Sciences* 110, no. 14 (2013): 5695–5700, http://www.pnas.org/content/110/14/5695.abstract.

444. "More Reasons Why Getting a Good Night's Sleep Is Important," *Newswise.com*, March 26, 2015, http://www.newswise.com/articles/view/631841/?sc=mwhn.

445. "Partial Sleep Deprivation Linked to Biological Aging in Older Adults," American Academy of Sleep Medicine, June 10, 2015, http://www.aasmnet.org/articles.aspx?id=5622.

446. Scott LaFee, "Women's Study Finds Longevity Means Getting Just Enough Sleep," *UC San Diego News Center*, September 30, 2010, http://ucsdnews.ucsd.edu/archive/newsrel/health/09-30sleep.asp.

447. "Sleep Duration Linked to T2DM Risk," *MPR*, June 18, 2015, http://www.empr.com/medical-news/sleep-duration-type-2-diabetes-risk/article/421445/?DCMP=EMC-MPR_DailyDose_cp&cpn=flecmpr, steld, xolderm&hmSubId=&hmEmail=LUGbza6izzVZv4gxnvu2QsU5jYgc1zdl0&NID=1700857323&dl=0&spMailingID=11674114&spUserID=MTgwMTYxMDE2MjI0S0&spJobID=561300963&spReportId=NTYxMzAwOTYzS0.

448. Janet M. Mullington, Norah S. Simpson, Hans K. Meier-Ewert, et al., "Sleep Loss and Inflammation," *Best Practice & Research Clinical Endocrinology & Metabolism* 24, no. 5 (2010): 775–784, http://www.bprcem.com/article/S1521-690X(10)00114-4/abstract.

449. "Snooze You Win? It's True for Achieving Hoop Dreams, Says Study," *Stanford Medicine News Center,* June 30, 2011, http://med.stanford.edu/news/all-news/2011/07/snooze-you-win-its-true-for-achieving-hoop-dreams-says-study.html.

450. Chris Woolston, "Sleep Deprivation and Stress," *HealthDay*, March 11, 2015, http://consumer.healthday.com/encyclopedia/stress-management-37/stress-health-news-640/sleep-deprivation-and-stress-646063.html.

451. "Napping Reverses Health Effects of Poor Sleep," *Newswise.com,* http://www.newswise.com/articles/view/629425/?sc=mwhn.

452. "Prolonged Shortened Sleep Increases Blood Pressure at Night, Researchers Find," *ScienceDaily*, March 13, 2015, http://www.sciencedaily.com/releases/2015/03/150313130739.htm?utm_source=feedburner&utm_medium=email&utm_campaign=Feed%3A+sciencedaily%2Ftop_news%2Ftop_health+%28ScienceDaily%3A+Top+Health+News%29.

453. "Impaired Sleep Linked to Lower Pain Tolerance," *Newswise.com,* April 30, 2015, http://www.newswise.com/articles/view/633488/?sc=mwhn.

454. "Severe Sleep Loss Affects Immune System Like Physical Stress Does," *Medical News Today*, July 2, 2012, http://www.medicalnewstoday.com/articles/247320.php.

455. "Napping Reverses Health Effects of Poor Sleep," *Newswise.com*, http://www.newswise.com/articles/view/629425/?sc=mwhn.

456. "Healthy Sleep Duration Linked to Less Sick Time From Work," *ScienceDaily*, September 3, 2014, http://www.sciencedaily.com/releases/2014/09/140903163633.htm?utm_source=feedburner&utm_medium=email&utm_campaign=Feed%3A+sciencedaily%2Ftop_news%2Ftop_health+%28ScienceDaily%3A+Top+Health+News%29.

457. "White Paper: Consequences of Drowsy Driving," National Sleep Foundation, http://sleepfoundation.org/white-paper-consequences-drowsy-driving.

458. "Drowsy Driving and Automobile Crashes," National Highway Traffic Safety Administration, http://www.nhtsa.gov/people/injury/drowsy_driving1/Drowsy.html.

459. "Circadian Rhythms Regulate Skin Stem Cell Metabolism and Expansion, Study Finds," *ScienceDaily*, January 6, 2015, http://www.sciencedaily.com/releases/2015/01/150106154607.htm?utm_source=feedburner&utm_medium=email&utm_campaign=Feed%3A+sciencedaily%2Ftop_news%2Ftop_health+%28ScienceDaily%3A+Top+Health+News%29.

460. "How Does Exercise Help Those with Chronic Insomnia," National Sleep Foundation, http://sleepfoundation.org/ask-the-expert/how-does-exercise-help-those-chronic-insomnia.

461. "Study: Physical Activity Impacts Overall Quality of Sleep," National Sleep Foundation, http://sleepfoundation.org/sleep-news/study-physical-activity-impacts-overall-quality-sleep.

462. "Yoga, Running, Weight Lifting, and Gardening: Penn Study Maps the Types of Physical Activity Associated with Better Sleep Habits," *Newswise,* June 4, 2015, http://www.newswise.com/articles/view/635242/?sc=mwhn.

463. Markham Heid, "You Asked: Is Sleeping in a Cold Room Better for You?," *Time.com,* November 26, 2014, http://time.com/3602415/sleep-problems-room-temperature/.

464. "What Is Keeping Your Kids Up at Night?," Stony Brook University Newsroom, September 4, 2014, http://sb.cc.stonybrook.edu/news/medical/140904kidsupnight.php.

465. Horacio O. de la Iglesia, Eduardo Fernandez-Duque, Diego A. Golombek, et al., "Access to Electric Light Is Associated with Shorter Sleep Duration in a Traditionally Hunter-Gatherer Community," *Journal of Biological Rhythms* 30, no. 4 (2015): 342–350, http://jbr.sagepub.com/content/30/4/342.

466. David C. Holzman, "What's in a Color? The Unique Human Health Effects of Blue Light," *Environmental Health Perspectives* 118, no. 1 (2010): A22–27, http://www.ncbi.nlm.nih.gov/pmc/articles/PMC2831986/.

467. "A Week's Worth of Camping Synchs Internal Clock to Sunrise and Sunset, CU-Boulder Study Finds," *BeBoulder.,* University of Colorado Boulder, August 1, 2013, http://www.colorado.edu/news/releases/2013/08/01/week%E2%80%99s-worth-camping-synchs-internal-clock-sunrise-and-sunset-cu-boulder.

468. Wilfred R. Pigeon, Michelle Carr, Colin Gorman, et al., "Effects of a Tart Cherry Juice Beverage on the Sleep of Older Adults with Insomnia: A Pilot Study," *Journal of Medicinal Food* 13, no. 3

(2010): 579–583, http://www.ncbi.nlm.nih.gov/pmc/articles/PMC3133468/.

469. Marian L. Evatt, "Vitamin D Associations and Sleep Physiology," *Sleep* 38, no. 2, http://www.journalsleep.org/ViewAbstract.aspx?pid=29854.

470. A. Slominski, T. W. Fischer, M. A. Zmijewski, et al., "On the Role of Melatonin in Skin Physiology and Pathology," *Endocrine* 27, no. 2 (2005): 137–148, http://www.ncbi.nlm.nih.gov/pmc/articles/PMC1317110/.

471. "Five Stages of Sleep," *Better Sleep, Better Life.com*, June 21, 2015, http://www.better-sleep-better-life.com/five-stages-of-sleep.html.

472. "What Happens When You Sleep?," National Sleep Foundation, http://sleepfoundation.org/how-sleep-works/what-happens-when-you-sleep.

473. "Five Stages of Sleep," http://www.better-sleep-better-life.com/five-stages-of-sleep.html.

474. Ibid.

475. Ibid.

Chapter 5: Rejuvenate Your Skin from the Outside

476. Makoto R. Hara, Jeffrey J. Kovacs, Erin J. Whalen, et al., "A Stress Response Pathway Regulates DNA Damage through β2-Adrenoreceptors and β-Arrestin-1," *Nature* 477 (2011): 349–353, http://www.nature.com/nature/journal/v477/n7364/full/nature10368.html.

477. "Antioxidants Cause Malignant Melanoma to Metastasize Faster," *ScienceDaily*, October 8, 2015, http://www.sciencedaily.com/releases/2015/10/151008131112.htm.

478. V. Lobo, A. Patil, A. Phatak, et al., "Free Radicals, Antioxidants, and Functional Foods: Impact on Human Health," *Pharmacognosy Review* 4, no. 8 (2010): 118–126, http://www.ncbi.nlm.nih.gov/pmc/articles/PMC3249911/.

479. L. E. Rhodes, G. Darby, K. A. Massey, et al., "Oral Green Tea Catechin Metabolites are Incorporated into Human Skin and Protect Against UV Radiation-Induced Cutaneous Inflammation in Association with Reduced Production of Pro-Inflammatory Eicosanoid 12-Hydroxyeicosatetraenoic Acid," *British Journal of Nutrition* 110, no. 5 (2014): 891–900, http://www.ncbi.nlm.nih.gov/pubmed/23351338.

480. Patricia K. Farris, "Resveratrol, the Longevity Molecule," *Dermatology Times,* April 30, 2015, http://dermatologytimes.modernmedicine.com/dermatology-times/news/resveratrol-longevity-molecule?page=0,0.

481. W. C. Quevedo, Jr., T. J. Holstein, J. Dyckman, et al., "Inhibition of UVR-Induced Tanning and Immunosuppression by Topical Applications of Vitamins C and E to the Skin of Hairless (hr/hr) Mice," *Pigment Cell Research* 13 (2000): 89–98, http://www.ncbi.nlm.nih.gov/pubmed/10841030; J. Y. Lin, M. A. Selim, C. R. Shea, et al., "UV Photoprotection by Combination Topical Antioxidants Vitamin C and Vitamin E," *Journal of the American Academy of Dermatology* 48 (2003): 866–874, http://www.ncbi.nlm.nih.gov/pubmed/12789176.

482. M. C. B. Hughes, G. M. Williams, P. Baker, et al., "Sunscreen and Prevention of Aging," *Annals of Internal Medicine* 158 (2013): 781–790, http://annals.org/article.aspx?articleid=1691732.

483. Frederic Flament, Roland Bazin, Sabine Laquieze, et al., "Effect of the Sun on Visible Clinical Signs of Aging in Caucasian Skin," *Clinical, Cosmetic and Investigational Dermatology* 6 (2013): 221–232, http://www.ncbi.nlm.nih.gov/pmc/articles/PMC3790843/.

484. D. H. McDaniel, I. H. Hamzavi, J. A. Zeichner, et al., "Total Defense + Repair: A Novel Concept in Solar Protection and Skin Rejuvenation," *Journal of Drugs in Dermatology* 14, no. 7 (2015): s3–11, http://www.ncbi.nlm.nih.gov/pubmed/26151795.

485. Lynne Peeples, "Study: Frequent Tanning-Bed Use Triples Melanoma Risk," *CNN*, May 27, 2010, http://www.cnn.com/2010/HEALTH/05/27/tanning.booth.melanoma/.

486. Jennifer R. S. Gordon and Joaquin C. Brieva, "Unilateral Dermatoheliosis," *New England Journal of Medicine*, April 19, 2012, 366e25, http://www.nejm.org/doi/full/10.1056/NEJMicm1104059.

487. Bruce Jancin, "EADV: Focus on Non-UV Triggers of Melanoma Risk Exposure," *Dermatology News*, December 11, 2016, http://www.edermatologynews.com/specialty-focus/skin-cancers-and-neoplasms/single-article-page/eadv-focus-on-non-uv-triggers-of-melanoma/67080c043b52aad7800cb5e6c4f085be.html.

488. Reena Rupani, "Probiotics for Healthy Skin," *Dermatology Times*, July 2015, 10, 18, http://dermatologytimes.modernmedicine.com/dermatology-times/news/probiotics-healthy-skin.

489. "Women Have More Diverse Hand Bacteria Than Men, According to CU-Boulder Study," CU News Center, University of Colorado Boulder, November 3, 2008, http://www.colorado.edu/news/releases/2008/11/03/women-have-more-diverse-hand-bacteria-men-according-cu-boulder-study.

490. W. R. Lee, S. C. Shen, W. Kuo-Hsien, et al., "Lasers and Microdermabrasion Enhance and Control Topical Delivery of Vitamin C," *Journal of Investigative Dermatology* 121, no. 5 (2003): 1118–25, http://www.ncbi.nlm.nih.gov/pubmed/14708614.

491. Heather Brannon, "Beta Hydroxy Acid," *About.Com*, http://dermatology.about.com/cs/skincareproducts/a/bha.htm.

492. D. S. Berson, "Natural Antioxidants," *Journal of Drugs in Dermatology* 7, 7Suppl (2008): s7–12, http://www.ncbi.nlm.nih.gov/pubmed/18681153.

493. Maeve C. Cosgrove, Oscar H. Franco, Stewart P. Granger, et al., "Dietary Nutrient Intakes and Skin Aging Appearance among Middle-Aged Women," *American Journal of Clinical Nutrition* 86, no. 4 (2007): 1225–1231, http://ajcn.nutrition.org/content/86/4/1225.

494. T. L. Duarte, M. S. Cooke, and G. D. Jones, "Gene Expression Profiling Reveals New Protective Roles for Vitamin C in Human Skin Cells," *Free Radical Biology & Medicine* 46 (2009): 78–87, http://www.ncbi.nlm.nih.gov/pubmed/18973801.

495. W. C. Quevedo, Jr., T. J. Holstein, J. Dyckman, et al., "Inhibition of UVR-Induced Tanning and Immunosuppression by Topical Applications of Vitamins C and E to the Skin of Hairless (hr/hr) Mice," *Pigment Cell Research* 13 (2000): 89–98, http://www.ncbi.nlm.nih.gov/pubmed/10841030; J. Y. Lin, M. A. Selim, C. R. Shea,

et al., "UV Photoprotection by Combination Topical Antioxidants Vitamin C and Vitamin E," *Journal of the American Academy of Dermatology* 48 (2003): 866–874, http://www.ncbi.nlm.nih.gov/pubmed/12789176.

496. "SkinCeuticals Unveils Novel Antioxidant Research," *SkinInc.com*, August 11, 2015, http://www.skininc.com/skinscience/ingredients/SkinCeuticals-Unveils-Novel-Antioxidant-Research-321418001.html#sthash.WolVa8Tt.dpuf.

497. "Lathering Up with Sunscreen May Protect against Cancer—Killing Coral Reefs Worldwide," *University of Central Florida Colleges & Campus News*, http://today.ucf.edu/lathering-up-with-sunscreen-may-protect-against-cancer-killing-coral-reefs-worldwide/.

498. Catherine St. Louis, "Night Creams in Sync with the Body's Clock?," *New York Times*, October 14, 2009, http://www.nytimes.com/2009/10/15/fashion/15Skin.html?adxnnl=1&adxnnlx=1384456596-SZcmZubasRg4Tf/DtsBBjA&_r=1&.

499. Linda W. Lewis, "Beyond Relaxing Lines," *MedEsthetics* 11, no. 6 (2015): 26–32, http://medestheticsmag.com/beyond-relaxing-lines.

500. Youn Sung Kim, Hyun Joo Lee, Sang Hyun Cho, et al., "Early Postoperative Treatment of Thyroidectomy Scars Using Botulinum Toxin: A Split-Scar, Double-Blind Randomized Controlled Trial," *Wound Repair and Regeneration* 22, no. 5 (2014): 605–612, http://onlinelibrary.wiley.com/doi/10.1111/wrr.12204/abstract.

501. Jim Kling, "Botulinum Toxin Injections Improve Depression," *MedScape*, March 26, 2014, http://www.medscape.com/viewarticle/822593.

502. T. S. Kuhnel, W. Shulte-Mattler, H. Bigalke, et al., "Treatment of Habitual Snoring with Botulinum Toxin: A Pilot Study," *Sleep Breath* 12, no. 1 (2008): 63–68, http://www.ncbi.nlm.nih.gov/pubmed/17882462.

503. S. J. Lee, W. D. McCall, Y. K. Kim, et al., "Effect of Botulinum Toxin Injection on Nocturnal Bruxism: A Randomized Controlled Trial," *American Journal of Physical Medicine & Rehabilitation* 89, no. 1 (2010): 16–23, http://www.ncbi.nlm.nih.gov/pubmed/19855255.

504. "SkinCeuticals Unveils Novel Antioxidant Research," *SkinInc.com*, August 11, 2015, http://www.skininc.com/skinscience/ingredients/SkinCeuticals-Unveils-Novel-Antioxidant-Research-321418001.html#sthash.WolVa8Tt.dpuf.

505. "The Science behind a Wrinkle Filler: Researchers Discover for the First Time How the Product Works," University of Michigan Health System Newsroom, February 19, 2007, http://www.med.umich.edu/opm/newspage/2007/restylane.htm.

9 780692 140338